REPRODUCING THE FUTURE

Marilyn Strathern and Janet Carsten
are series advisers
for Manchester University Press's
publishing in Social Anthropology

REPRODUCING THE FUTURE

Essays on anthropology, kinship and the new reproductive technologies

Marilyn Strathern

Manchester University Press

Published by Manchester University Press
Oxford Road, Manchester M13 9PL, UK

British Library cataloguing-in-publication data
A catalogue record for this book is available
from the British Library

ISBN 0 7190 3673-9 *hardback*
0 7190 3674-7 *paperback*

Printed in Great Britain
by Bell & Bain Limited, Glasgow

CONTENTS

PREFACE

This volume marks an epoch of sorts. The essays belong to, and the majority were written during, the time when the Bill for the Human Fertilisation and Embryology Act (1990) going through Parliament had stimulated public debate in Britain. The implications of the medical developments that lay behind the Act are world-wide. These essays touch on the British debate from the particular perspective of an anthropologist.

New procreative possibilities – fertilisation *in vitro*, gamete donation, maternal surrogacy – formulate new possibilities for thinking about kinship. At the same time, and inevitably, possibilities are imagined through ideas already in existence and already part of a cultural repertoire. As cultural facts, such ideas inform our representations, descriptions and analyses of kinship, and the future of kinship lies in their future too. The same issues also open up larger questions about how to think the interaction between 'nature' and 'culture' as such. Anthropologists have their own investment in the concept of culture, and questions are in turn raised about how anthropology will reproduce its concepts in the future.

My hope is that together the essays will demonstrate one kind of contribution that anthropological knowledge can make to current debate. It is knowledge that openly draws on substantive materials from other parts of the world, and hence from other people's cultural facts, even when it is most about home. Thus the present essays are informed by recent rethinking of models of kinship in Melanesia. This serves as a reminder of what is at stake in fashioning new descriptions of kin relations. Anthropological knowledge offers a transparent example of the process involved in rethinking through concepts and images whose expressible forms already belong to other repertoires and thus to other specific domains of ideas. In that it borrows as much from itself and its own past as it does from elsewhere. And in that sense the world is kin.

People everywhere express or communicate even the most general of thoughts in specific and particular forms; indeed they make their ideas available to one another through such forms. As a consequence they are always borrowing, if only from themselves. It is this (cultural) facility that enables us to at once give shape to and provide ourselves with starting points for fresh thought.

ACKNOWLEDGEMENTS

My gratitude to various publishing bodies for being allowed to reproduce material already or about to be in print is background to the list below. In addition, I thank those facilitators who held, convened and/or otherwise organised the occasions which made me write these chapters in the first place: their names are given on the title pages to Parts I, II and III.

Janet Carsten's interest in the new kinship has been a stimulus to my thinking. I also owe a collective debt to my colleagues in the Department of Social Anthropology at Manchester University for enabling me to take a term's research leave in 1991, and in particular for Tim Ingold's and Frances Pine's assistance. Discussions with Andrew Holding have been a pleasure, as has been receiving comments from Nigel Rapport and Erica Haimes.

Many of the papers were reworked (and Chapters 7 and 8 written) with the specific interests of a research project in mind: I am grateful to the Economic and Social Research Council for the award (ROOO 23 2537) for an exploratory study into The Representation of Kinship in the Context of the New Reproductive Technologies. The other members of the research team are already part of the present enterprise, and my gratitude is self-evident. In addition, Jeanette Edwards's investigations have been an inspiration; Sarah Franklin furnished me with many ideas; Eric Hirsch paced me with his own Melanesian/English balance; and Frances Price has been a friendly and trenchant critic – I hope I have not blurred too many of the issues she sees with such clarity.

Richard Purslow proved a proactive editor of the best kind, while my thanks to Jean Ashton continue to accumulate. Karen Egan has been a magnificent support when I have been distracted from other things. And for appearing not to mind other gaps in what could have been a more ample enactment of kinship, I thank Barbara, Hugh and Alan.

Apart from differences in footnoting conventions, and with the exception of Chapter 1 for editorial reasons, the papers are printed here virtually as they will have appeared elsewhere. Notes are at the back of each chapter where relevant, clarifications for the present edition being indicated by asterisk in the text itself. Each is thus a self-contained piece: where some of them draw on the same material, I ask the reader's interpretative indulgence. Cultural facts never just replicate themselves – they are forever recontextualised, 'borrowed' indeed, and perhaps the repetitions will have the effect of reproducing substance in ways that never take quite the same form.

I am grateful to the publishers concerned for permission to use material which has appeared in the following.

Chapter 1   Sage, London, *Changing Human Reproduction: A Social Science Perspective*, to be edited by M. Stacey

Chapter 2   The Editors, *Cambridge Anthropology*, 14: 1–12, 1990; and Unwin Hyman, London, *The Values of the Enterprise Culture – The Moral Debate*, eds P. Heelas and P. Morris, 1991

Chapter 3   Edinburgh University Press, *The Age of the City*, eds A. Cohen and K. Fukui [in press]

Chapter 4   The Editor, *Australian Feminist Studies*, 10: 49–69, 1989

Chapter 5   Routledge, London, *Conceptualizing Society*, ed. A. Kuper, 1992

Chapter 6   The Editor, *New Literary History*, 22: 581–601, 1991

Chapter 7   [not previously published]

Chapter 8   Routledge, London, *Contemporary Futures*, Association of Social Anthropologists Monograph series, ed. S. Wallman, 1992

Marilyn Strathern, Manchester, May 1991

INTRODUCTION

Artificial life

'You start with a living thing and you start taking it apart and you see what parts it has and how all these parts fit together and try to derive some general principles of the logical organisation of those parts. It's OK up to a point, but you take ... it apart further and all of a sudden you don't have life any more, life sort of slips through your fingers.'

'In a sense what we're working on is an alternate form of biology, because it's a sort of might have been biology. One problem with biology is we only have one example of an earth having evolved ... We're using the computer to simulate imaginary biological worlds and we say "what if", and we can do experiments that would really be impractical to do in a real biological system.'

This interchange took place on a British television programme screened in the summer of 1990 (Wyver 1990); the two American speakers, Chris Langton (Los Alamos National Laboratory) and Danny Hills (Thinking Machines Corporation) were discussing artificial life. They offered a contrast between traditional biology that could only 'get a handle on what life is' through analysis – taking things apart to observe the composition of characteristics – and the possibilities afforded by computer simulation. Here one can synthesise various characteristics to observe the effect of combining them.

As the second speaker said: 'The alchemist's dream was that you mix together the right combinations of elements and suddenly a creature will emerge out of it and talk with you. In a sense what we're doing is not so different from that, but instead of mixing together chemicals, we're mixing together programmes and bits of information and the soup is a soup that lives inside a computer.'

There is something about these imaginary worlds that would interest a social scientist. The speakers – experts in their field – bring together characteristics or properties to make new models that will have properties of their own, including the capacity for replication which turns them into 'life forms' of a kind. And the way the experts *describe* what they are doing has similar properties: they bring together concepts and images. They do this when they evoke different worlds (the new scientist is both like and not like the alchemist) or draw on metaphors that convert the uncommon to the common (analysis is seeing) or draw on analogies that spell out a relationship (being in the situation of analysing deeper and deeper is like being in the situation of taking something apart till nothing is left). As an imaginative activity, this bringing together is verbally summed up in the hybrid idea that gives its name to their enterprise: artificial life.

Such combinations are not so different from what is presented daily in advertising. They depend on a balance between the synthesis that produces a novel entity and the analytical differentiation of elements without which the combination would not be visible. Think of 'intelligent building', for instance, a Japanese architect's description of office blocks in Osaka: the new idea works because buildings are not otherwise thought of as having intelligence. Or what Mitsubishi do with concepts when they describe an organic car ('organically inspired vehicles ... cars that perform as an extension of your will') under the heading 'Created as living hardware'.[1] The adjectives summon an image that refers to a whole different world from what would otherwise be associated with the product in question, a domain of ideas that does not 'naturally' belong to it.

Here are deliberate extensions of the facility for making analogies that is central to cultural life anywhere. Indeed, what constitutes a natural or logical domain of ideas gives an image its cultural stamp. This is equally true of what is thinkable in terms of combinations and syntheses – you can tell a culture by what it can and cannot bring together. Take an example from kinship. In some parts of the world it is regarded as proper to express affection between relatives through making payments to them; it is expected that these activities will be linked. In other parts of the world commerce and kinship are held separate; here the one activity cannot be expressed through the other without raising questions about their very character. Now what is thinkable with respect to kinship has a particular interest of its own.

It has become routinely thinkable in the post-industrialism of the late twentieth century – or at least presentable in Euro-American[2] media – to make play with juxtaposing images of the organic and inorganic. We are not just supposed to think that machines are like bodies, but that there are aspects of machines that function no differently from parts of the human body even as human beings may embody technological devices within themselves. The one does not imitate the other so much as seemingly deploy or use its principles or parts. An established parallel already exists in the way the relationship of biological to social life is described in terms of a contrast between what is natural and what is artificial or socially constructed. The parallel lies in kinship thinking. Kinship systems and family structures are imagined as social arrangements not just imitating but based on and literally deploying processes of biological reproduction.

While Euro-Americans have become aware that particular forms of kin arrangements are specific to particular cultures and societies, and artificial in that sense, it is taken for granted they are there to deal with the natural facts of life. These natural facts are thought of broadly as biological or more narrowly as genetic. The idea of a genetic parent, for instance, brings together what is known about human heredity and the fact that a relationship is entailed, since for Euro-Americans it is virtually impossible to talk of a parent in a human context without evoking the idea of potential social relations.

Now if culture consists in established ways of bringing ideas from different domains together, then new combinations — deliberate or not — will not just extend the meanings of the domains so juxtaposed; one may expect a ricochet effect, that shifts of emphasis, dissolutions and anticipations will bounce off one area of life onto another. And while culture is a world of the imagination, it is not a fantasy one whose power lies in the impossibility of realisation. On the contrary, it has its constraints and its effects on how people act, react and conceptualise what is going on around them: it is the way people imagine things really are.

One might, then, ponder upon how to think about experiments being conducted in a real system that is regarded as *both* a biological *and* a social one — what constitutes kinship for Euro-Americans. I do not refer to scientific experimentation in the narrow sense, though it was the need to formulate regulations under which research on human reproductive material was acceptable that led (among other things) to the legislation recently enacted in the British Parliament. I mean experiment in a larger sense. Developments in reproductive medicine have made it possible to intervene in the procreation of children in unprecedented ways, and under conditions where the full implications can only be known through the outcome of the intervention itself. Thus a further stimulus to legislation concerned one outcome already in existence: the fact that a potentially new legal and social entity had come into the world in the form of the human embryo in the very early stages of development, alive but outside the parental body. How to think it, that is, imagine it and make it real, became a matter for debate. This was also true of the general idea of 'reproductive technology', an already existing set of interventions already pressed into service.

Background debate

The passing of the British Human Fertilisation and Embryology Act in 1990 was an occasion for such debate. Quite apart from the parliamentary discussions themselves, the issues that led to the formulation of the Act were assumed to be in the public mind. Indeed, the earlier Committee of Inquiry led by Mary Warnock, an initial exploration of what should be taken into account in legislation, had been called to respond to, if not actually allay, public concern. For many people in Britain, the concern was with the kind of future that might follow increasingly sophisticated techniques of intervention in the reproduction of human life. 'Technology' suggested a future of more, not less, recourse to what 'it' could do.

Debate never gathered together in one place; nonetheless, differences of public opinion became evident in relation to one another. Thus the knowledge and interests of those directly involved in research or in clinical practice sometimes appeared juxtaposed to what they saw as the public misunderstanding of science or as unfounded nightmare scenarios, as well as to the overt needs of those for whom such developments offered hope and relief. We might say that here was a society reflecting on the implications of some of its own capabilities. What kind of cultural awareness did people bring to bear on the issues?

The essays that follow record the cultural education forced on an anthropologist encountering some of these issues for the first time and largely via the popular media (press, television, public conferences). While this route might have led to an awareness of a particular and limited nature, it had properties that are generalisable.

Awareness takes shape against previous experiences, earlier positions, interests formulated for other purposes and other contexts. Thus (new) ideas are thought through other (old) ideas. What already exists may well be sedimented in common values and institutions, and in what people take to be the moral thing to do. After all, morality presumes that, even if not demonstrably shared by them, principles are at least applicable to others. It is also exemplified in modes of conceptualisation, in practices of thinking, in habits of speech – in short, in cultural facts. Habitual images and familiar metaphors provide the cultural forms that make ideas communicable.

At times, forms long taken for granted may come under a challenge that seems sudden or unprecedented. There is a challenge of this kind in these late-twentieth-century debates. And that is precisely because, in addressing the processes of procreation, they address what twentieth-century 'English'[3] culture had *taken for granted* as the foundation for relations between kin and for the formation of family life. Now the family is a more colloquial and familiar category than kinship (the English simply assume that families are composed of persons who are kin to one another). However, the concept of 'kinship' allows me purchase of a particular kind.

By kinship I understand not just the ways in which relatives interact with another, but how relationships as such are held to be constituted. Having sex, transmitting genes, giving birth: these facts of life were once taken as the basis for those relations between spouses, siblings, parents and children which were, in turn, taken as the basis of kin relations. Incorporated into such a reproductive model were suppositions about the connection between natural facts and social constructions. These ideas about kinship offered a theory, if you like, about the relationship of human society to the natural world. They also incorporated certain ideas about the passage of time, relations between generations and, above all, about the future.

It is no accident that thinking about intervention in this area should bring futuristic fantasies and (in some cases) doom-laden scenarios to some people's minds. For the intervention is also into ideas, including ideas about the future itself – what it is that we are laying or seeding for generations to come.

Such futures necessarily belong to the present: they are what we imagine for ourselves now. The present is itself only made visible against a past, and if I have used a past tense to describe certain ideas, it is not because people no longer think them but because the range of other ideas with which they can think them has altered. It is impossible to measure the range, just as it is impossible to enumerate all the different positions in a debate that is, so to speak, society-wide. Yet it is possible to provide something of a description of how we might imagine ideas having a range. We would be looking at the diversity of domains that particular images traverse.

These essays were never intended as a direct contribution to the debates stimulated by the then Bill. Rather, they come from the side, and in doing so individually exemplify a principal message of this book as a whole. They point to an outcome of the domaining effect. In cultural life, in those habits of thought about which for most of the time we are very much unaware, the ideas that reproduce themselves in our communications *never reproduce themselves exactly*. They are always found in environments or contexts that have their own properties or characteristics. These environments or contexts provide a range of domains. We can think of all the social differences that opportunity, class, gender, expertise and so forth make to how the world is perceived; interests such as these form several such environments, and profoundly shape the nature of communication. Moreover, insofar as each is a domain, each imposes its own logic of 'natural' association. Natural association *means* that ideas are always enunciated in an environment of other ideas, in contexts already occupied by other thoughts and images. Finding a place for new thoughts becomes an act of displacement.

But one may well ask who 'we' are and in whose culture the new reproductive technologies intervene (cf. Seal 1990). I point to the question rather than answer it. The unanswered question, then, is as to what and whose views will get re-sedimented in publicly promoted discourse, including future legislation.

A significant limitation of my position should be noted. In drawing on various media interpretations of concern raised by new reproductive technology, especially as stimulated by the parliamentary debates and the kind of evidence available to the Houses of Parliament at the time, my very rendering of the issues is contextualised in a particular way. The media interpretations were themselves re-rendering the kind of 'scientific' knowledge on which public knowledge draws. In this, they offered a set of cultural facts from a prominent domain of consumer culture. However, this re-rendering and these cultural facts do *not* represent public opinion at large, let alone contemporary biological thinking, nor even reflect what many people take for granted in their kinship practices. A case in point emerges in the crucial role that certain specific and specialised perceptions of individuality played in the definition of personhood for those considering the status of the early embryo. Several of the chapters that follow dwell on this issue, since the representation of individuality became a preoccupation of its own.

Such perceptions of individuality have general cultural saliency. But they inevitably displace further ways of representing persons. Here we see how, with particular intentions, including the most pragmatic of reasons, people draw from certain domains of ideas to the exclusion of others. Thus the relational[4] and familial concerns that many English people additionally hold, and that may be voiced in respect of procedures involving (say) donation or surrogacy, have seemed irrelevant to the scope of legislation. They have only found their way into the official debate through an allowance for the 'need' of the child or the counselling needs of those involved in treatment. We might say that broader relational and familial concerns constitute something of an indigenous anthropology.[5] Certainly they provide an alternative voice; and certainly they call for empirical attention. Such alternatives are, however, no more than noted in this book.

The present volume

In having been written for a specific audience, each of the essays that follow offers its own focus. Perhaps one can capitalise on the multiple perspectives of topic and intention, for perspectives are also vantage points and theoretical positions may indicate social ones; a note is made, at least, of the original reason for writing.

The position reproduced here is that of an anthropologist who was a student during the heyday of what was called British Social Anthropology (see Chapter 5), and whose theoretical interests have since been shaped by feminist scholarship and, above all, by Melanesian ethnography (Chapter 4). Over the last thirty years, the societies of that part of the world have given anthropologists much to think on − and to rethink as far as their own premises are concerned. The chapters in Part III make this apparent. While my particular understanding of the Papua New Guinea Highlands (and especially Hagen) remains in the background, I inevitably draw on a recent synthesis of some of that rethinking (Strathern 1988). Equally in the background is a brief experience working with English materials from an Essex village; here rethinking has been of a different kind (Strathern 1992). The second exercise was not driven by quite the same desire to make sense of puzzles and contradictions in anthropological arguments about the nature of social life as in the Melanesian case, for such a breadth of argument does not yet exist in anthropological work on Britain. It was instead fuelled by a desire to find a way of reacting to the cultural revolution of (as it was then) British Thatcherism.

Reaction implies engagement of a kind, and the initial chapters (Part I) were first given to non-anthropological or mixed audiences. Indeed, Chapter 2 stemmed from a conference on the values of the Enterprise Culture; it is a reaction to the value we nowadays award 'choice'. When choice has such a cultural platform, it comes to seem problematic, even in the context of enlarging people's reproductive options. For by the end of the 1980s, the Enterprise Culture had turned coagulant, like a slick that smothers everything in shine. I vent my prejudice at the outset. It is a prejudice tempered through having to live the cultural revolution in one's workplace, where students are supposed to mean numbers, public accountability must be interpreted as resource management, and education has to appear as a service for customers. The rest of the book is an attempt to mediate the prejudice by criticising the cultural revolution anthropology-fashion: to make its new analogies work for how we might think old problems. As already noted, however, my sources put a specific limit on the exercise.

The cultural revolution is, of course, far wider than the Enterprise Culture, which I take as a cheap and nasty version[6] of what is more interestingly thought in other modes. It goes elsewhere under such cataclysmic rubrics as the End of Modernity or, more ambiguously, Postmodernism. If for much critical practice it means the demise of the author as individual subject,[7] for the anthropologist it brings uncertainty to conceptualising that counterpart to the individual, namely 'society'. Similar uncertainties attend the parallel antonym between 'nature' and 'culture'. In commenting on the way the concept of nature is drawn into the representation of fertility treatments, Chapter 3 speculates on whether the concept of culture might have a future.

The question of how one might think the relationship between nature and culture is broached right at the beginning (Chapter 1). This offers another kind of speculation. Part of the shine on the Enterprise Culture comes from defining services as provisions responsive to customer preference. In this mode, fertility treatment can be seen as a service facilitating people's exercise of options in the face of natural needs.[8] Chapter 1 asks what is means to assist kinship in this way. It shows how the rooting of social relations in natural facts is made evident in assumptions about the individuality of persons and the recognition of biological ties. The original venue for the essay was the British Association meetings for 1990, and the same meetings provided a story that introduces Chapter 6.

Part II constitutes a break of sorts. What up to this point have been general comments on changing cultural practices, as they might appear to an anthropologist reflecting on the values and analogies of culture-at-home, are shown (in my case) to have a background in feminist interests on the one hand and Melanesian ethnography on the other. The still less-than-easy relationship between these two components in my thinking is laid out in Chapter 4. The same chapter also introduces the reader to a body of ethnography.[9] The purpose is to offer at least one extended example of the possibilities afforded by Melanesian materials, since elsewhere my references are sketchy. It also (briefly) makes concrete a contrast with an American study, which again provides at least one location for ideas that are elsewhere in this book presented at a remove from their social contexts.

Neither Chapter 4 nor 5 refers to the new reproductive technologies. They are concerned instead to provide a theoretical context for those ideas of person and relationship that inform Euro-American – and English – kinship practice. Both were written for specialist audiences, and contain allusions to arguments internal to feminist or anthropological debate. Thus Chapter 5 takes up the challenge of a postmodern critique of the concept of culture in order to think back on conventional anthropological wisdom concerning the nature of Euro-American kinship. It touches on conceptualisations of personhood, body and generation in both Euro-American and Melanesian societies that supposedly typify cognatic systems.

The essays that make up Part III each lay out a direct contrast between aspects of Melanesian thinking and aspects of Euro-American ideas about kinship. They return to issues in the new reproductive technologies raised earlier. But whereas Part I is concerned with certain general ways in which to frame some of the cultural implications of change in this area, the final chapters address specific points of debate. They have a unity in that they all touch on discussions concerning the status of the early embryo. I add that the focus is mine, and although a significant preoccupation it was by no means the only one in the public mind.

Chapter 6 concerns the concept of donation, as in the donation of gametes (ova and sperm). Comparison with Melanesia comes into its own here, for anthropologists have long described relationships there as premised on gift exchange. But the comparison is cautionary, and the point of the chapter is to reinstate the Euro-American 'gift' in the context of the values of individualism and consumer culture which is also the context for contemporary ideas about kinship. If it rediscovers what Titmuss argued many years ago in *The Gift Relationship*, I let the rediscovery stand for the possible interest that the different route took. It explores, for example, the implicit analogy between an individual's relationship to society on the one hand and an organism's relationship to its environment on the other.

Most analogies drawn in this book are offered as interpretive moves on my part. Chapter 7 was stimulated by an analogy evoked explicitly and deliberately in part of the debate on embryology in the House of Lords. This leads to a reflection on the relationship between social interpretation and natural fact, and how this composite is replicated in ideas both about the embryo itself and about motherhood and surrogacy. It dwells on the concept of development, at once enabling of debate and troublesome to it.

Development is integral to the anticipation of what organisms might become: Chapter 8 continues with arguments concerning the early embryo, in this case outside Parliament. It returns to some of the specifications of individuality raised in Chapter 1. Although its purpose is to draw a lesson for the way anthropologists might wish (or not wish) to anticipate the future of their subject, it also shows that in taking decisions about the nature of the embryo, at least some of the contributors to this particular debate found themselves drawing on concepts from different domains and thus on widespread and generally shared formulations. At the same time, such formulations acquire in turn their particular forms by the contexts in which they are deployed and carry different resonances in different domains of expertise. Indeed, they never carry over from one to another exactly.

This makes evident one of my starting points: that it matters what ideas one uses to think other ideas (with). Reproduction concerns everyone. Yet when human beings reproduce themselves, they inevitably do so with already existing and thus specific forms of themselves in mind.

Notes

1 Both examples are from publications aimed at the English-speaking world. The first comes from a description of an optical fibre network laid down by National-Panasonic for an office block in Osaka built with 'the information-intensive society of the 21st century' in mind. Environment, office automation, communications, audio-visual technology: 'The intelligent office building is an organic integration of these four concepts'. The second example comes from an advertisement for the Mitsubishi Galant, from an in-flight magazine of Japan Airlines, April 1990.

2 The hybrid is preferable to the monolithic 'Western', though needs further specification as North American/Northern European. Contemporary Japanese culture may or may not contribute to this discourse.

3 'English' is used in this volume to index specific cultural practices; the fact that one could as well substitute other, though not identical, specificities (e.g. North American, Scottish) makes the point. Elsewhere I have accounted for a hegemonic reading of 'English' as middle-class, literate, and a source from which many taken-for-granted academic theorisings come. ('British' refers to the inhabitants of Britain, that is, to a population and a state not to a culture.)

4 One of my intentions in drawing contrasts with Melanesia is to show how difficult Euro-Americans find it to conceptualise relationships. Melanesians take relationships for granted, as vital supports for all living persons, and work to differentiate persons from one another. Euro-Americans take individuality as basic to a natural condition, so that 'relating' persons to one another is itself a kind of cultural enterprise, even when one is looking for natural relations. As a consequence, their ideas about kinship give priority to individualism. It might appear, then, as though I am advocating an 'individualistic' approach. I am not. Rather, I wish to show how ingrained the representation of individualism is in certain areas of discourse in order to show that it is (like 'nature') a cultural artefact. There are alternative discursive possibilities in Euro-American practice, of which the anthropological representation of Melanesia serves as a reminder. The 'otherness' that Melanesians occupy in this account is addressed briefly in Chapter 4 (also see Chapter 8); Strathern (1991) suggests a way in which Melanesians conceivably anticipate a postmodern future.

5 Anthropology is committed to a relational view on technical grounds insofar as its practice lies in making relations explicit (though for the nostalgia possibly in store for it, see Strathern 1992).

6 Sir Peter Swinnerton-Dyer's reported characterisation of the ethos under which he had to lead the Universities Funding Council (Wojtas 1991: 2) ['cheap even if it is nasty'].

7 This might seem to present a paradox. In fact, one can read the hyper-individualism of the Enterprise Culture as the other side of the coin to the death-of-the-individual in some postmodern aesthetics.

8 A trenchant comment on the creation of need in this area is given in Morgan and Lee (1991: 165).

9 Thanks to Sarah Franklin for suggesting I include this essay.

PART I

Chapter 1 As 'The Meaning of Assisted Kinship', this originally contributed to Margaret Stacey's President's Day, Section N (Sociology), at the 1990 meetings of the British Association for the Advancement of Science

Chapter 2 'Enterprising Kinship: Consumer Choice and the New Reproductive Technologies' was first given to a conference on 'The Values of the Enterprise Culture', convened in 1989 by Nicholas Abercrombie, Paul Heelas, Russel Keat and Paul Morris at Lancaster University

Chapter 3 'Future Kinship and the Study of Culture' was presented at 'The Age of the City', a symposium held by The Senri Foundation during Osaka's 1990 celebrations for the 21st century; the symposium organiser was Katsuyoshi Fukui

CHAPTER 1

Kinship assisted

At the 1987 meetings of the British Association, a speaker in the Psychology section asked why the concept of kinship in human beings was a problem. Wells was commenting on the way non-human animals modify their behaviour on the basis of relatedness to other members of their species. Tadpoles can apparently tell the difference between siblings, half-siblings and unrelated individuals, while some bees behave as though they can distinguish 14 degrees of relatedness. Human beings have similar facilities: mothers are able to distinguish their own infant from others by cry within 48 hours of birth, and by smell within a few days. However, in her view, the problem that human beings create is that their *ideas* about kinship do not match directly on to the facts of biological relatedness. 'We don't perform kin recognition in the way that animals do because we have the concept of kinship' (Wells, reported text of BAAS paper, Belfast).

Biological relatives, the speaker stated, are those with whom we share genes by descent. But we also 'recognise' other people as relatives who are not really relatives; 'aunt', she says, is often used to refer to people 'who are not really aunts'. The paper then went on to reveal the discovery that despite the kinds of concepts people hold about their kin, biologically related kin are often given preferential treatment. The author drew on a theory of kin selection that is much contested. Nonetheless, these themes (kinship, relatedness, biology) were of enough moment to be reported at length in the quality press (*Guardian*, 28.8.87).

As in other areas of scientific enquiry, discoveries in social science may follow the pattern of this one, bringing to light fresh facts about behaviour. But there are also those kinds of discovery that do not unearth fresh facts so much as make fresh connections. The present exercise falls into the second class. It explores some of the ways connections are made between facts, and does so in the light of an anthropological assumption about cultural practice.

The anthropological analysis of culture points to the general human facility for making ideas out of other ideas. We make fresh concepts by borrowing from one domain of life the imagery by which to structure other areas – as Darwin apparently did by finding in nineteenth-century ideas about degrees of kinship and affinity the vocabulary for his nascent theory of natural selection (Beer 1983). But images pressed into new service acquire new meanings. Thus the idea of affinity between species gives fresh resonance to the idea of human affinity. Old meanings in turn are destabilised, and indeed the whole process may generate uncertainty. Hence the *Guardian* prints a story on kinship because changing practices in family relations mean we are not quite certain what to borrow or where to borrow from, the appropriate analogy to draw. Perhaps tadpoles and bees will help. But how we seek help already gives a shape to the problem.

Reproductive medicine is no exception. I suggest that the way in which changes in this field are conceptualised, and the way the choices that assisted reproduction affords are formulated, will affect thinking about kinship. And the way people think about kinship will affect other ideas about relatedness between human beings. What follows is a brief demonstration of connections between various aspects of kinship as they were aired at the time of the passing of the Human Fertilisation and Embryology Act (1990). It pretends to analyse neither the parliamentary debates themselves nor the public debate as it was carried on in the press and in other publications, nor indeed does it presume that there is only one debate. Instead, it illustrates some common cultural strategies in the communication of concerns. The concerns address formulations about the nature of kinship that characterises British society. Broadly, one may think of these formulations as 'Western' or Euro-American insofar as they are recognisable across Northern European and North American cultures; narrowly, one may think of them as belonging to specific forms of middle-class consciousness and enquiry, of interest in this country insofar as they provide the language in whose terms evidence came before Parliament and was filtered back to the public via the press.

Pritchard, a geneticist, recently complained about the way people are screened from scientific knowledge in reproductive medicine. Instead of being given the responsibility of making decisions for themselves, legislation makes it necessary for them to seek expert advice. Often this will be medical even though the issues surrounding the example he cites – surrogacy – are not medical but ethical and legal. What is interesting is that he borrowed an analogy from education: people learn, he is reported as saying (*Daily Telegraph*, 7.4.90), through participation rather than formal instruction. This makes a connection for his observation that 'ethical problems are problems for individuals, not legislation' (Pritchard, Meeting on Genetics and Society, University of Leicester). He thus used an assertion about learning to make an assertion about freedom of choice. It is exactly the manner in which he thus borrows one set of ideas (education) to talk about another (freedom) that enables me to make a counter-assertion. I shall also make connections, but of a different kind.

The statement about legislation seems to me misplaced. Ethical problems are problems for society, because of – among other things – the way they draw on and simultaneously challenge existing ideas about human life.

Biological relatives

Darwin drew on the prevailing ideas of his time concerning genealogy and relatedness between human beings in order to depict degrees of affinity between other species. In the twentieth century Euro-Americans have turned this back on itself, and conceive biological relatedness as primordial and prior to the constructs human beings build upon it. People even talk of biological relatives.

In ordinary parlance, a 'relative' means a kinsperson, that is, one whose degree of relationship is socially recognised. The whole point of Wells's paper was that non-human animals do not recognise kinship. So to talk, for instance, about siblings in other species is to repeat Darwin's loan: the idea of a relative is borrowed from the affairs of human beings. But we also see how this becomes a two-way traffic, since the idea of biology is borrowed in turn to depict an essential or intrinsic component of relatedness between human beings. Biological relatives, Wells claimed, are not only those who share genes but they are the 'real' relatives. Real relatives, her argument adds, are likely to exercise choice and preference on one another's behalf.

This two-way traffic of ideas makes the concept of kinship a hybrid of different elements. Human kinship is regarded as a fact of society rooted in facts of nature. Persons we recognise as kin divide into those related by blood and those related by marriage, that is, the outcome of or in prospect of procreation. However, the process of procreation as such is seen as belonging not to the domain of society but to the domain of nature. *Kinship thus connects the two domains.* This is a combination that Euro-Americans reproduce several times over in their ideas about relatedness between human beings, and it is such reproduction and repetitions that constitute cultural practice.

Let me give an example. Family life is held to be based on two separable but overlapping principles. On the one hand lies the social character of particular arrangements. Household composition, the extensiveness of kin networks, the conventions of marriage – these are socially variable. On the other hand lie the natural facts of life. Birth and procreation, the inheritance of genetic material, the developmental stages through which a child progresses – these are naturally immutable. To talk about 'kinship' is to refer to the manner in which the social arrangements are based on and provide the cultural context for the natural processes. Indeed, such an overlap of concepts supports the prevailing twentieth-century orthodoxy in much anthropological and other social science approaches to culture, namely that the subjects of study are 'social constructions'. In the case of kinship, what is at issue is the social construction of natural facts. At the same time, established critiques, including those from anthropology, make it evident that what are taken as natural facts are themselves social constructions (see Franklin 1991). What is revealed is another hybrid.

It is important to realise that this cultural practice – the way in which ideas from different domains are brought together – is not just the preserve of social scientists and their theories of social constructionism. It is endemic in Euro-American habits of thought. The Human Fertilisation and Embryology Act stipulates that a woman shall not be provided with treatment services unless account has been taken of the welfare of the child-to-be, including the child's need for a father. Now, as it was reported at the time (e.g. *Guardian*, 21.6.90), the need for a father was justified during the course of the House of Commons debate by reference to a domain of social fact that had nothing to do with relatedness and only tangentially bore on the child's development. The mover of the amendment in question was reported as arguing that we tinker at our peril 'with the concept of the family being a financial unit which needs two people'. He thus brought together two different domains of experience, establishing the focus of concern (here the family) by overlapping criteria. Families constitute relationships produced by procreation on the one hand and household or financial organisation on the other.

The example shows something else. Connections are motivated. The importance of the father's presence is being justified by implicit reference to housekeeping and income support. The concept of the family as a financial unit thus grounds the argument about fathers. One could equally well imagine the reverse conceptual strategy: a reference to the desirability of maintaining children's relationship with their fathers grounding an argument about income support and taxation.

This kind of cross-referencing is so habitual that one hardly stops to think about it. But it plays a significant part in people's views of the world. What the speaker was grounding was a sense of reality. One set of ideas under dispute (whether or not the 'need' for a father should be part of treatment screening) is grounded in another set whose reality at that juncture is not questioned. At that juncture, the idea of the family as a financial unit needing two people is not under debate, precisely because it is being deployed as a taken-for-granted point of reference.

In the concept of biological relatives or in the idea of kinship as the social construction of natural facts, the biology and the natural facts are taken for granted. Euro-Americans do not ordinarily dispute what these are. Indeed, they may be colloquially unspecific.

Finch's (1989) recent investigations into patterns of family obligation in Britain came up time and again against the special place that people gave to 'blood' ties. The character of family life and kin connections is frequently grounded by reference to this domain of nature. The concept of a blood 'tie' symbolises the further fact that relatives are seen to have a claim on one another by virtue of their physiological make-up. With respect to understandings in social science, Finch discusses competing theoretical claims over whether 'biology is at the centre of mutual support in families' (1989: 218), including kin selection theory (in this latter view, people are likely to favour their own 'because of the biological relationship between them'). But however disputed the theories, and whether one is thinking as a social scientist or not, everyone seems to take it for granted that *a biological relationship has significance for human affairs.*

The idea of a biological relationship does double symbolic service. As a taken-for-granted reference point, it is one way of grounding the distinctiveness of kin relations. But it itself also indicates what can be construed as immutable or taken for granted in the human condition: the natural facts of life that seem to lie prior to everything else.

An anthropologist would argue that to sustain a domain of ideas as a reference point is also to sustain its separateness. The 'difference' between domains is affirmed in their being brought into relation – as when one supplements the other. Hence reference to the family as a financial unit introduced a fresh dimension to the debate on parents. In the same way, to think of kinship as the social construction of natural facts at once combines and separates the domain of social affairs from the natural world. Neither dimension will entirely substitute for the other; both are necessary, and the difference between each is sustained.

Individual kin roles within Euro-American kinship systems repeat this overlap. Each plays out the hybrid combination in microcosm. An unambiguous kinsperson is both related by blood *and* is one whose relationship is acknowledged in forms of intimate care. Schneider (1968) formalised this division for American kinship by talking of the distinction between substance and code for conduct. A mother both gives birth and nurtures her child; you share genes with your mother's sister, but she enters your life as an aunt because of the visits and presents. As a result, there may be a problem where the overlap does not completely hold, when one element but not the other seems present, as in the case of in-laws. I doubt whether our ancestors of (say) 200 years ago were troubled in quite the same manner. It is very much a post-Darwinian problem.

In twentieth-century culture, nature has increasingly come to mean biology (cf. Ingold 1986). In turn this has meant that the idea of natural kinship had been biologised. What is to count as natural has acquired rather specific meanings. And one challenge that the new reproductive technologies hold is how they will affect these meanings in the future. Already they have introduced into regular parlance the distinction between 'social' and 'biological' parenthood. Now biological parenthood does not replicate with exactness the old concept of natural kinship. It reproduces the idea. But, in reproducing the idea, it also introduces a new difference.

There is a new ambiguity about what should count as natural. The 'natural' father was once the progenitor of a child born out of wedlock; the 'natural' mother was once the progenitor of a child relinquished for adoption. Ideally the social parent combined both biological and legal credentials, though it was not ordinarily necessary to mark the parent in this way. Contemporary possibilities of artificial procreation introduce a new contrast between artificial and natural process: assisted reproduction creates the biological parent as a separate category. By the same process, the social parent becomes marked as potentially deficient in biological credentials. (Glover (1989: 57) refers to '*either* the social *or* the biological father' (my emphasis).) The effect is thus a displacement of earlier usages. So the 'natural' parent of the future, if one may extrapolate, may well turn out to be the one for whom no special techniques are involved and the one on whose behalf no special legislation is required. In that case it would be the natural parent who combined both biological and social/legal attributes.

Insofar as kinship is thought of as combining social and natural domains, and is thus the place of overlap between them, the recognition of one component without the other always gives people pause. What is new is the assistance being given to each domain. The natural facts of procreation are being assisted by technological and medical advances. The social facts of kin recognition and relatedness are being assisted by legislation. Kinship is doubly assisted. There is a further outcome to such assistance, for it takes away the very concept that made kinship itself a distinctive domain. There is little now to be taken for granted.

Assisting the making of persons

Treatments available for remedying 'impaired' fertility make explicit the widely shared cultural assumption that persons desire children of their own.

Now while the origin of genetic material has consequences for the person born of it, and is part of his or her identity, conception is held to depend neither on that identity nor on the relationship of the couple. It is thought to be a (natural) process that operates independently of human intention. Human intention gets no further than acting on the desire itself. I make the remark apropos Euro-American thinking on the matter and with certain very different kinship systems in mind. In Melanesia, for instance, much cultural effort can be expended on making sure that persons conceive in the right relational context: infertility may be attributed to deficiencies in social relations, and facilitation will then attend to people's intentions in the matter. By contrast, Euro-Americans find nothing exceptional in the possibility of facilitating the physical process, an operation regarded as independent of personal or social identity.

The paradoxical outcome is that facilitating the process does not automatically assist the making of parents. It assists the making of children, but then the English word 'child' means both offspring and young person. What is assisted is the making of persons, and specifically individual persons.

Debates concerning embryo experimentation reveal an interesting combination of ideas surrounding the creation of new human life. With whatever caution Parliament and the government's Committee of Inquiry (Warnock 1985) had approached this topic, there is no doubt many assumed that the 'central question of when a human being came into existence' (*Guardian*, 24.4.90) was the issue. This entailed a further assumption. Life was seen to inhere in living cells, humanness in the fact that they are produced from human genetic material. But the point at which 'a human being' could be said to have emerged was presented as the point at which the *individuality* of the physical matter that will make up the future body and mind of a single entity could be discerned. With the establishment of the individual, in this view, comes a necessary condition for the establishment of the person, that is, an entity with potential moral claims on others. Yet those claims seem a consequence of, rather than a cause of, its personhood (and cf. Smart 1987). No relationship with other persons, not even its parents, affects the way the issue of personhood is generally discussed.

There was considerable dispute as to what demarcates that individuality. It might be said to be a divine spark that sanctifies life from the 'beginning' of fertilisation. It might be said that embryos at a developmental stage prior to brain formation and consciousness are not persons. The potential rather than actual consciousness of the embryo became an area of contest and controversy.* However, whether people talked of a soul or of a mind, the presumption was that they were talking of a quality existing in the singular (e.g. Ward 1990: 110: 'a person is a subject of rational consciousness'). Yet, as Dyson (1990: 99) remarks, as far as ethics are concerned one should

---

* The location of one version of this debate and some of the arguments are detailed in Chapter 8.

also consider the possibility that the ethical unit cannot be the individual as such, for human beings exist only in interdependence with other human beings. This was not an issue that found easy formulation. It is interesting to consider why.

From one perspective, the answer is trivial: the parliamentary debate concerned embryos first, of which their status as potential persons was a secondary attribute; the legislation was not about defining persons. But, from another perspective, the absence fits certain general cultural suppositions that affect the way people think about kinship.

First, Euro-Americans tend to visualise interdependence in the abstract, and can imagine a person without reference to other persons. Thus the adult individual may well be described as dependent 'on society'. They do not use dependence on relatives to stand for interdependence in general (embeddedness in kin relations will not do as a symbol for membership in the wider society). Instead they try to conceptualise interdependence through abstract and universal criteria such as common humanity or interaction between an organism and its environment [see Chapter 6]. Dyson refers to an 'interdependent human community' rather than to the interdependence of specific persons.

Second, Euro-American ideas of individuality are grounded in notions of physical discreteness. Thus the House of Commons allegedly made up its mind about the admissability of embryo experimentation by focusing on the '14-day limit'. Its significance was spelled out by reference to biological process. 14 days is just before the so-called primitive streak can be seen, the precursor of a specific and single embryo: 'the rubicon is crossed between molecular matter and a potential human being' (Morgan and Lee 1991: 68). At the same time, two 'clearly defined populations of cells' are apparent, those that will form the embryo and those that will form the placental support system (1991: 68). The chair of the then Interim Licensing Authority is quoted as saying that the formation marks 'the beginning of a unique, human individual' (*Daily Telegraph*, 23.4.90). At least, this was one of the forms in which biological information was conveyed to those debating the Bill.*

---

* Because knowledge in this field is advancing at such a fast rate, the information that came to the House was not only translated for a lay audience but inevitably contained already out-of-date formulations, that in turn 'mixed' with formulations already held (e.g. the idea that fertilisation could be said to have a beginning).

However controversial the particular limit, the *significance of individuality was not disputed*. The central question of when 'a human being' came into existence was answered unanimously: when one can recognise a unique individual. At a yet later stage one might start to talk of a human personality or person. Indeed, if the issue of personhood had nothing to do with interpersonal relationships, it had everything to do with developmental stages. Now once an individual person is born, his/her needs and rights inevitably exist in relation to those of others, and the very necessity to legislate on such needs and rights comes from the fact that persons are never isolated from the actions, effects, presences of others. But, in this dialogue conducted with respect to the being not yet born, the emergence of personhood itself was taken to be a natural process, the outcome of biological development rather than the person's own moral standing or participation in relationships with other persons.

So what becomes the issue at debate is the stage of growth.* While other persons may act on behalf of the person-to-be as though it were already born, the embryo/foetus does not respond with a presence of its own. Or rather, its personhood is anticipated above all by reference to its physical presence. Of course action is taken on behalf of non-responsive entities all the time (Gallagher 1987), as it is on behalf of persons with immature or impaired responsiveness. Nonetheless, it is of some moment, I think, to imagine the very reproduction of persons in a non-relational way.

Like kinship, in the Euro-American view, individual persons are commonly construed as a hybrid of the two dimensions referred to earlier. On the one hand persons always inhabit a social and cultural world of which they are actively part and which they help create; on the other hand they exist as naturally individual beings with needs and desires of their own. The dimensions overlap when the person is thought of both as a member of society and as an autonomous individual whose existence is defined by other criteria such as physiological and developmental processes. But there is also an asymmetry here. Indeed, the latter may be prioritised over the former: the one dimension (individuality) acts as a grounding and reference point for the other (personhood).

* An interesting critique of this term is considered in Chapter 7.

Assisting the making of parents

Discussions surrounding the prospects of assisted reproduction make explicit the fact that no one comes into existence without the joining of complementary substances. One cannot exist without having parents.

It is an axiomatic tenet of Euro-American kinship reckoning that everyone has parents in this biological sense, whether or not one knows who they are. For the simple transmission of the substances themselves is thought to confer identity. Self-consciousness about identity in turn is interpreted as part of the individual's rights as a person: thus the child's 'right to know' the origin of its genetic make-up has been an important part of the debate ever since the Warnock Report (1985). But the interests of parents and children may conflict, and knowledge does not necessarily lead to a relationship.

The child's right to know inevitably raises the question of its relationship to its 'biological parents'. It is from the consequences of such revelation (it was commonly argued) that those who donate reproductive material, but who do not wish to be known as parents, should be protected. In other words, what might be good for the child is not necessarily good for the parents. A different conflict emerges in the evaluation of parental involvement in the child's upbringing, for a further axiom of Euro-American kinship is that parents must give their children the right environment. Biological parenting and social parenting are thus combined again in the idea that the fitness of social parents turns on their ability to provide the proper natural circumstances for the child to grow up. The focus here is on the child's needs both as a developing organism and as an individual self with a psycho-emotional profile, so the parents become defined in relation to its perceived needs. It is assumed that these may compete with other aspects of the parents' lives as persons. Indeed, generally in Britain, the duties of parents to children are more clearly acknowledged than the duties of children to parents (see Finch 1989). Inheritance aside, since duty and responsibility fall on the parent with respect to the child, it is assumed that parenthood should be recognised in law. But the law finds itself acknowledging biological parenthood even where one might have thought its business was the definition of social parenthood.

A distinction between social and legal recognition is traditional. The former concerned the acknowledgement of a relationship, the latter rights in law. Thus the Glover Report can consider the case of Swedish law, where the semen donor is socially recognised in that the child (at age 18) has a right to know who he is but he has no rights of legal paternity in the child. The implication is that it is desirable to match legal paternity to social rather than biological paternity as far as the family in which the child will grow up is concerned. 'Social parenthood often out-ranks biological parenthood ... And the emotional bond with the social father is usually far more important to children than the genetic links with the donor' (Glover *et al.* 1989: 35). The social relationship, however, is still being justified in reference to a biological process of sorts, the process being a universal one concerning the child's needs as a developing human being. So while a social parent is given preference over a biological parent, the significance of the social parent is once again established by reference to a non-social aspect of development. In this imagery, 'the relationship' does not exist between persons, then, so much as between the mutuality of their natural needs.

Debates over who shall be regarded by society as parents, then, are *not* the mirror image of debates over the beginning of life. And that is because of the priority that the biological facts of life have in grounding the very perception of the 'real' situation. Hence the asymmetry to which I referred. Thus the discussion over human beginnings proceeds without reference to social factors at all: when a person begins is taken as a biological fact of individual development. By contrast, the legal debate over who shall be socially acknowledged as parent makes constant reference to biological parenting: legislation is after the fact.

The reason for this asymmetry rests in the two points already made. First, it is possible to conceive of a child as having claims on society directly and in its own right. Its relationship with its parents is enabling for personal development, but its claims as a full moral and legal individual are on society in general rather than on its parents in particular. Parents only mediate this future relationship and, if necessary, society in the person of the state can intervene to protect the child's welfare. Second, the individuality of persons is imagined in terms of their uniqueness (physical discreteness) as functioning organisms. A person's social life is regarded as extrinsic: in interactions with others the individual person is influenced or affected by them, but such interdependence frequently appears negotiable. People become parents because parents are said to want children of 'their own'. The colloquialism, an interesting fusion of whom one identifies with and what one owns against the world, points to desire or preference. The child has no choice as to which parents are its own, but may prefer to escape their influence or spurn their property: it is the person's individual status not its relationships which guarantee its own personhood.

As a result, attempts to define relationships, such as that between parent and child, render the actual notion of relationship elusive. On the one hand, Euro-Americans make the maintenance of relationships dependent on the preference of persons (e.g. 'in the end ethical decisions are made by taking into account human preference', Ward 1990: 112), which echoes the remark quoted at the beginning (the idea that ethical problems are problems for individuals). Persons, as we have seen, are thought of as individual subjects. On the other hand, insofar as social arrangements are regarded as constructions on natural facts, themselves perceived as above all biological facts, people feel that definitions of relationship should incorporate and pay attention to these facts. Social relationships appear contingent. These points connect two versions of the same construct. Biology is rooted in an order of reality to which social arrangements must attend, not the other way round.

We are used to this asymmetry in the definitions of 'mother' and 'father'. The two are not mirror images of each other either. The division between what we now see as biological and social parents, or between the biological and social identities of any single parent, is also reproduced in the division between the evidently biological involvement of the mother with her child and the necessity to presume and therefore socially construct fatherhood. Even where what is at issue is the father's biological contribution, that is popularly supposed to depend on social acknowledgement in a way a mother's parenthood is not.

Sections 27 and 28 of the British Human Fertilisation and Embryology Act determine the 'meaning of "mother" ' and the 'meaning of "father" ' in certain cases of assisted conception. The woman who is the carrier of the child is in law to be treated as the mother. The explanatory notes to the Bill added, 'whether or not the child is genetically hers'. As far as the father is concerned, the Act provides for the husband of a married woman who has conceived through donation to be treated in law as the father of the child so long as he consented to the donation. This follows the recommendation of the

Warnock Report, in relation to which Rivière (1985) pointed out some time ago that the intention to treat a person *as* a mother or father implies that this is a social construction (a legal 'fiction') on the natural facts. In this case, the natural fact is that he is not the biological (genetic) father. Commentators (Morgan and Lee 1991: 154–6) interpret the protection of anonymity afforded sperm donors as, in the absence of any consent from a husband or other man, creating a legally 'fatherless' child. It is not that a real father (the genetic father) does not exist, but (as they see it) that the law forbids his being socially acknowledged.

In the past, the natural facts that define a mother always seemed more comprehensive than those defining her partner. She both donated genetic material and brought the child to term, elements combined in the former cultural assumption that childbirth was a supreme natural fact of life. Now the period of gestation has become culturally ambiguous, and in the new division between biological and social motherhood, the mother's nurturing role shifts from being regarded as part of a total biological process to being the principal attribute of a social one. At the same time, the very conceptualisation of artificial or assisted conception means that the pre-birth process is no longer a definitive natural fact either.

In Western (Euro-American) middle-class culture, parenthood traditionally presumed a relationship between persons. Yet there was a constant lopsidedness or asymmetry to the depiction of relationships for the very reason that they appeared to be constructed after natural facts. The converse was the supposition that if there is a biological tie, then there is always the question of whether or not social recognition should follow. Yet current legislative attempts to define who shall be the parent, when faced with a range of choices, introduces an explicitness that may make the *fact* of relationship more rather than less uncertain. Being donor of reproductive resources, provider of gestatory facilities, postnatal nurturer – as separate elements none is sufficient ground for acknowledging the connection as a relationship. A decision has to be taken on what kind of social relation is desirable as a consequence of the biological one.

In making a new convention, the distinction between social and biological parenting, out of an old one, kinship as the social construction of natural facts, the new reproductive technologies have provided unprecedented alternatives for legislation. Legislation in turn creates new explicitness. The Glover Report, a document suffused with an ideology of preference and choice, is hopeful that 'our ability to separate social from biological parenthood may create new patterns of relationship' (1989: 53). I suggest three outcomes over which we may have little cultural choice.

First, the chances are that we shall go on trying to accommodate the representation of relationships to what is perceived as their natural basis – whether in biology at large or in genetics. The justifications and representations will change as fast as our views of the facts change. Given the determining role we accord to the biology, how we represent those facts to ourselves will thus affect us all.

Second, while social relationships appear to respond to and deal with biological facts, from an anthropologist's point of view those facts are also cultural facts, constructs that are themselves socially or culturally motivated. We are in something of a new area when they become legally motivated. Which points of law are going to apply to the management of the natural world can be expected to play an increasingly significant part in our lives. Even being able to conceive of life forms as subject to patent, offers intriguing analogies for the proprietorship of persons.

Finally, the rooting of social relations in natural facts traditionally served to impart a certain quality to one significant dimension of kin relations. For all that one exercised choice, it was also the case that these relations were at base non-negotiable. The idea of a blood tie symbolised their given nature. There was a matter-of-factness to them that did not just concern the performance of kin obligations, important as that was. Ties of kinship in general stood for what was immutable about one's social circumstances by contrast with what was open to change. In being urged these days always to exercise preference and choice, we may find ourselves acting out a curious version of those kin selection theories, to which Wells briefly referred and which themselves incorporated a version of Euro-American kinship thinking. Selecting what relatives one chooses to keep up with is one thing; selecting one's parentage is another.

The fatherless child

This brings me back to the manner in which we assist ourselves. In effect, Euro-Americans are being forced to be explicit about aspects of their own social and cultural practices in attempting to meet the needs they perceive.

In the same year as Wells's address, a short article appeared in the journal *Free Associations* on 'The crisis of fatherhood'. Its questioning of the notion of fatherhood is modelled by way of analogy on that of motherhood: 'Who is the father? Is he the man who provides the sperm ... or the man who cares for the child?' (Smith 1987: 72). The choice of the word 'care' rather than 'provide' was apparently deliberate, for the author attempts to put (social) fathering on the same nurturant footing as mothering. What prompts Smith's question is the issue of artificial insemination. It is not that assisted procreation is new, then, but that it has entered the cultural repertoire in a way as to make such questions relevant to *any* conceptualisation of parenthood.

Not surprisingly, Smith finds that fathers and mothers are not mirror images of each other. In asking about the emotional weight men put on biological fatherhood he discovers that their physical involvement cannot match women's: 'I as a man have not become pregnant, nor borne a child, nor am I breast-feeding one with my body milk. Unlike a woman, I am not *physically* tied to any one child once conception occurs' (1987: 75, original emphasis).

The implication seems to be that emotional bonds flow from physical ones. As a result, doubts (his term) can be expressed at every stage, for at every stage there are new doubts about the physical ties. There are doubts about the relevance of male sexuality to conception, about the fact of genetic fatherhood, about the desirability of cohabitation, about how one manages emotional needs and the practicalities of child care and male labour. Doubts about the physical ties are doubts about relationships. In essence, this self-analysis takes apart an already established combination of social and natural relations. Break the parental role down into its components, and at no point does there seem an essential connection between the physical person and the social relationship of parent to child. Smith suggests this is particularly true of men. Women, not men, tend to take responsibility for contraception, he says; women are more certain than men of their biological parenting, women seem able to dispense with cohabitation as a precondition for bringing up a child, and so forth. But the comparisons he makes are merely one instance of a whole series of cultural connections between what is certain and what is uncertain in kinship arrangements, a version of the connection repeated over and again between natural–biological and social–legal parenthood.

The doubts remain real, and point in one direction. Unless a relationship is grounded in some intrinsic or natural connection, then Euro-Americans are likely to think of it as artificial, and to be thought artificial is to be open to uncertainty. Reality must lie elsewhere.

The new reproductive technologies and the legislative and other actions to which they have given rise seek to assist natural process on the one hand and the social definition of kinship on the other. But this double assistance creates new uncertainties. For the present cultural explicitness is revolutionising former combinations of ideas and concepts. The more we give legal certainty to social parenthood, the more we cut from under our feet assumptions about the intrinsic nature of relationships themselves. The more facilitation is given to the biological reproduction of human persons, the harder it is to think of a domain of natural facts independent of social intervention.

Whether or not all this is a good thing is uncertain. What is certain is that it will not be without consequence for the way people think about one another.

CHAPTER 2

Enterprising kinship: consumer choice and the new reproductive technologies

There is, we are told, an argument 'for letting the future shape of the family evolve experimentally. No doubt people should be discouraged from taking high risks ... And it goes without saying that new forms of family life must only be tried voluntarily. But subject to these qualifications, we *prefer a society* predisposed in favour of "experiments in living" to one in which they are stifled' (Glover *et al.* 1989: 63, my emphasis).

Thus the Glover Report on Reproductive Technologies to the European Commission. The committee was asked to consider ethical and other social issues raised by the techniques that (as they put it) 'extend our reproductive options' (1989: 13). By reproductive option they mean primarily fertility, although their concern extends from artificial insemination, *in vitro* fertilisation and 'maternal surrogacy' to future implications of gene therapy and embryo research. They suggest that these new techniques will enable us to influence the kinds of people who are born. Indeed, the techniques are bracketed together under the opening observation that perhaps our time will be seen as 'the era when we became able to take control of our own biology, and in particular to take control of our own reproductive process' (1989: 13).

But what are we supposedly taking control of? What is being reproduced? In many cultures of the world, a child is thought to embody the relationship between its parents and the relationships its parents have with other kin. The child is thus regarded as a social being, and what is reproduced is a set of social relations. At the least, the child reproduces parents' relational capacities in its own future capacity to make relations itself, as often indicated for instance in marriage rules. Yet the future that the Glover Report holds out to us, with its benign language of voluntarism and preference, is rather different. What is apparently at stake is the fate of human tissue, and what these techniques will reproduce is parental *choice*. The child will embody the desire of its parents to have a child.

Consequently, conflict of interest is expressed as a matter of who wants what. Hence the brief discussion of donor anonymity turns on what the donating man 'wants' and whether or not the social parents will 'want' their family complicated by a relationship with the biological father (1989: 24). Again, the question of surrogacy contracts turns on the couple 'wanting' the child to be healthy, 'wanting' to end the relationship with the surrogate mother (1989: 69), and so on. In the language of desire, the question of rights turns on the right to fulfil what one wants, and in a much larger way that is the justification for the enabling technologies. They help persons fulfil themselves.

This has for long been a significant if unremarkable cultural motivation, in both Britain and Europe, for having families. The point is that the kind of people on whose opinions the Glover Report drew now see themselves in a world that is developing technologies specifically enabling of this desire. That potency can eclipse or summate the diversity of factors that lead to children being born. Hence the equation between reproduction and fertility: what is 'extended' is the choice to have children.

Extending the choice

I put it thus to draw attention to certain elements contained in such ways of presenting ourselves to ourselves. And to get away from the idea that these ideas about having children only affect the having of children. For there is a kind of tunnel vision to much of the discussion that assumes that all that is at issue is childbearing, and that the only people concerned are those who have personal problems to solve. However, I am not addressing the capacity of any of us to have or not have children, and nothing of what I say either approves or denigrates those whom the technologies aid. My direction is elsewhere.

By 'ourselves' I do not claim to speak on behalf of contemporary British society, but simply to identify myself with those who are exposed − whether they wish for it or not − to a range of ideas and images now in cultural currency. One does not have to be governed or preoccupied by such ideas in order to be aware of their significance; it is sufficient that they have been conceived, expressed and thus made available as vehicles for further ideas. The issue, then, is not whether these technologies are good or bad, but with how we should think them and how they will think us. The issue is the forms of thought they present through which we shall look on other aspects of human affairs, such as kin obligation, nurture, friendship and so forth.

Glover and his associates make a gesture in that direction: they state that the problems raised by the new reproductive technologies 'require a response by society as a whole' (1989: 15). By this they mean what framework of law should exist: how far 'should these decisions affecting the future of the family and affecting which people are born, be left to emerge from the decisions of individuals or couples, and how far should there be a deliberately planned public policy'. Society's intervention is thus thought of as endorsing public opinion of the form of policy measures, and the policies will be about parents and children ('the family' in their account is simply a parent-and-child group). Yet it is a rather narrow view of everything we might wish to think of as pertaining to society to bundle it all up in policy measures, as it is an extraordinarily impoverished view of culture to imagine that how we conceive of parents and children only affects parents and children.

Culture consists in the way analogies are drawn between things, in the way certain thoughts are used to think others. Culture consists in the images which make imagination possible, in the media with which we mediate experience. All the artefacts we make and the relationships we enter into have in that sense 'cultural' consequences, for they give form and shape to the way we think about other artefacts, other relationships. A simple example: the Report draws on a contrast between rigidity and flexibility in order to contrast two sets of opinions. While one can imagine contexts where either quality might be preferable, built into the contrast is a preference for flexibility − extension is good for its own sake. The metaphor imparts a concreteness to the contrast between opinions. We draw on such metaphors all the time.

It is because we do this all the time that the issues here are serious. The new reproductive technologies (hereafter NRT) are presented as opening up reproductive options, indicating a vision of a biology under control, of families free to find their own form.

However fantasised these images of future choice are, it is also the case that in the name of enlarging the possibilities of human fulfilment, techniques are refined, medical advice is given, and we hold on to the hope that human beings will only find benefit from genetic engineering (e.g. Ferguson 1990). A phantasia of options on the one hand and actual decisions being implemented on the other. However one looks at it, procreation can now be *thought about* as subject to personal preference and choice in a way that has never before been conceivable. The child is literally — and in many cases, of course, joyfully — the embodiment of the act of choice.

Yet not just the children born by such techniques: so also those not born by them, and so also those not born at all. Glover *et al.* notice in passing: 'Not to make these choices will itself be a choice' (1989: 56). They do not refer simply to the decision to have a child; by this stage in the Report they are referring to the future possibility of determining sex and other genetic characteristics.

Perhaps there is nothing remarkable about all this, except for one thing. Until now, it has been part of most of the indigenous cultural repertoires in Europe to see the domain of kinship, and what is called its biological base in procreation, as an area of relationships that provided a given baseline to human existence [see Chapter 1]. Kin relations, like genetic make-up, were something one could not do anything about. More powerfully, when these relations were thought of as belonging to the domain of 'nature', nature also came to stand for everything that was immutable, that was intrinsic to persons or things, and as those essential qualities without which they would not be what they were. It is not just that kin relations were regarded as constructed out of natural materials, but that the connection between kinship and the natural facts of life symbolised immutability in social relations.

By now my point must be obvious. What do we do with the idea that a child embodies its parents' wishes, that families will find whatever form their members desire, that kinship might no longer be something one cannot do anything about? How will this all work as an analogy for other relationships? If till now kinship has been a symbol for everything that cannot be changed about social affairs, if biology has been a symbol for the given parameters of human existence, what will it mean for the way we construe any of our relationships with one another to think of parenting as the implementing of an option and genetic make-up as an outcome of cultural preference? How shall we think about what is inevitable and not really open to change in relationships, a question that bears on the perception of people's obligations and responsibilities towards one another.

Parents as customers of parenting services? Biology under control? Customers respond to a market, not to 'society'; biology under control is no longer 'nature'. Shall we find ourselves bereft of analogies – shall we no longer be able to 'see' nature, or 'see' society for that matter? For if kinship and procreation have been understood as belonging to a domain of nature, if nature has in turn symbolised what we have taken as inevitable constraints on the conduct of social life, then society by contrast has been thought about as human enterprise working on these givens, and thus a realm of endeavour carved *out of* the natural world. If the givens of our existence vanish, by what shall we measure enterprise? But I go ahead of myself. Let me remain with the fact that we now live in a world where alongside whatever other thoughts one had about parent–child relations must come the thought that the child ought to exist by choice. In this world the idea of choice is already embedded in a matrix of other analogies.

This matrix is the Enterprise Culture. As the report to the European Commission indicates, it is a culture more widespread than its particular manifestations in Britain. Nevertheless, it is useful to draw on Keat's (1990) account of the British version.

The value given to preference and choice in decision-making over the NRT already reveals the workings of analogy on analogy. Those who seek assistance, we are told, are better thought of not as the disabled seeking alleviation or the sick seeking remedy – analogies that also come to mind – but as customers seeking services. The new technology, meanwhile, enables persons to achieve desires that they could not achieve unaided. However, a further enablement is required to take advantage of the services (cf. Pfeffer 1987): money is literally enabling of the enabling devices. We can think of these services not just as human enterprise being exerted on behalf of those who wish to be enterprising, but as a business that caters to those who will make a business out of being a family.

Yet there is something about the market analogy that is less than benign. It tends to collapse all other analogies into itself, the effect being rather like that of money itself which, in differentiating everything makes itself the only source of difference. For instance, Keat refers to the collapse of the distinction between production and consumption when production is consumer-led and when consumption becomes a business itself. This reverses the normal order we imagine that production takes, that you first find out what can be sold and then make it. Yet more than reversal is at issue. What worked about the dialectic between productive consumption and consumptive production was that each term was a reference point for the other, a given point of departure, whereas what seems to characterise the present dispensation is that we are unwilling to cede such stable reference points because of the particular one that we privilege. The producer manufactures according to the consumer's choices, and the consumer purchases according to the choices the manufacturer lays out. Choice has become the privileged vantage from which to measure all action. Yet choice is by definition destabilising, for it operates as much on whim as on judgement. That at least is the cultural vision.

Consumers and producers live alike by one another's choices. In fact, we could say that producers turn out the embodied choices of their customers, and consumers choose among the embodied choices of those who provide the services. One glimpses a world full of persons embodying the choices of others. Perhaps one day we shall find some way of being able to reproduce the choices without the bother of putting them into bodies.

The absurdity offers the real glimpse of a situation where choice might cease to be enablement. In fact we could have made that connection long ago. If we are to look for what is 'rigid' about the Enterprise Culture, for what stifles enterprise, for the new givens of our existence, it lies in the hidden prescription that we *ought* to act by choice. This is not sophistry; it is a point of political concern.

Prescribing the choice

Not everyone has been tunnel-visioned about the NRT. Notable exceptions are found in the works of feminist scholars, and many of my observations simply remake observations already made (for a recent review, see Franklin and McNeill 1988). There is the question of prescriptive fertility, for instance, that accompanies what one could call prescriptive consumerism, namely the idea that if you have the opportunity to enhance yourself you should take it. Feminists are aware of pressures put on persons to appear to be fulfilled in certain ways. For, in the Enterprise Culture, one's choices must always be self-enhancing, the catch being that the self and its enhancement will only be recognised if it takes specific forms (Rose 1991).

Thus Pfeffer (1987) asks why, in the late twentieth century, personhood has become equated with the capacity to reproduce, almost to the point of the difference between the fertile and infertile becoming analogous to that between the donors and recipients of charity. New techniques of 'fertilisation' do not remedy fertility as such, but childlessness; they enable a potential parent to have access to the fertility of others. A new divide between have and have-not is implied, insofar as technology has already opened up to personal choice the 'decision' to have children. The enterprising self, as Keat says, is not just one who is able to choose between alternative ways, but one who implements that choice through consumption (self-enhancement) and for whom there is, in a sense, no choice *not* to consume. Satisfaction is not in this rhetoric the absence of desire, but the meeting of desire. To imagine an absence of desire would be an affront to the means that exist to satisfy it.

The sense that one has no choice not to consume is a version of the feeling that one has no choice not to make a choice. Choice is imagined as the only source of difference: this is the collapsing effect of the market analogy. Like the Warnock Report (1985) before it, the Glover Report goes out of its way to comment on commercialisation in transactions involving gametes. One can think of reasons why commerce is discouraged. Yet the point is surely that the market analogy has already done its work: we think so freely of the providing and purchasing of goods and services that transactions in gametes is already a thought-of act of commerce. All that rearguard action to protect the idea of the family from the idea of financial exploitation, to reconceive such transactions as altruistic or acts of love or as real gifts between persons, are after the event – these ideas have no other ideas to fall back on. If kinship is to be an enterprise like anything else, then where are the relationships that will enable us to think of gamete donation as a gift? Glover *et al.* say that in 'families and between friends, gifts are more common than sales' (1989: 88). But gifts pass between friends and kin precisely to indicate the non-transactable part of their relationship. With whatever nuance of taste or sentiment, one gives to express a solidarity or celebrate a relationship that once in place has no choice about it. If the idea of a gift sounds hollow or off-key in reference to gamete transfer, it is because the Enterprise Culture provides many more and readier ways of thinking about a calculating self.

Enterprising culture

Prescriptive consumerism dictates that there is no choice but to always exercise choice; its other side is prescriptive marketing. Culture is being enterprised-up.

I was once − naively − appalled meeting a colleague (from another profession admittedly) who cheerfully announced being on the way to the library in order to 'scholar-up' a paper, to add the references that would make it look scholarly. Naively, because I had imagined scholarship was in the nature of the product. Now in exercising their choices, consumers are concerned both with product identity and with product identification. The exercise of choice that defines the active citizen is market choice, not just because of the kinds of rules of the game associated with free bargaining or an equation between enterprising selves and business enterprises, but because the market deals in things which have been market*ed*. That is, they are designed for selling, made to specifications that anticipate consumer wants, presenting back to the consumer 'choice' in the form of a range of products out of which 'choice' can visibly be made. To choose repsonsibly, our active citizen must know what is being offered, much of this knowledge being filtered through appearance: things must look what they are supposed to be. Apples must look like apples. One might say they have to be appled-up; varieties are selected for marketing which have the most apple-like qualities. Qualities essential to the realisation of choice become displaced, as it were, from the product onto what is presented for the consumer's discrimination.

Marketed products are quality-enhanced. Quality is not there to be discovered: those attributes which define things are made explicit, even superadded, in the course of the marketing process. Marketing does much of the selection for you, and consumer activism is generally in the area of greater determination over what the producer claims to present. So one selects for quality where quality means both an innate characteristic (firmness, taste) and an enhanced version (unblemished flesh, shiny skin). The term 'quality' has always had this ambiguity. But the marketing of products forces an interesting collapse of its two senses. The natural, innate property and the artificial, cultural enhancement become one. To select an apple for its appleness is to discriminate between those which conform more and those which conform less to cultural expectations about what the natural apple should be. Glover *et al.* raise the question of whether handicapped people and those born with physical blemish can have a totally fulfilled life.

There is a little more at stake here than one might think. This is not a new essentialism but a collapse of the difference between the essential and superadded. The market*ed* apple is 'the apple and a bit more', that is, a fruit that will attract the consumer for its appleness. What is collapsed is the difference between what is taken for granted in the nature of the product and what is perceived to be the result of extra human effort.

Although in referring to apples I have, so to speak, natured-up my example, the same point can be made with respect to manufactured articles, for whether utilitarian or luxury their qualities are enhanced by the efforts of advertiser and marketeer. Indeed, they are not 'marketable' without 'extra' attention being drawn to their 'inherent' characteristics. It is of some further significance that what we take as the domain that stands for what is natural, inherent and so forth in human affairs is not immune from an elision of a similar kind.

Among various models for human affairs that have held sway over the last 200 years has been a distinction between the taken-for-granted in human relationships and the culturally constructed, between the natural individual and the society that socialises the individual into its own mould. This is one of many such binarisms that has moulded the development of social science and is arguably where our model of enterprise comes from – its natural parents, if you like. In this model, human beings are enterprising creatures who 'construct' and made what they will 'out of' the givens of existence and environmental constraints. We would thus contrast enterprise, that is, culture or society in the twentieth-century sense, endless variety testifying to an endless igenuity, with other factors that appear given, immutable, universal, of which biological reproduction, like sexual difference, has till now been a prime example.

The contrast between human ingenuity (enterprise) and natural constraints is replicated in microcosm in European thinking about kinship. Anthropologists in the European tradition argue that there are many different ways in which cultures enterprisingly construct families and type of kin relations, but of course human beings everywhere are dealing with the same raw material, the facts of nature: of procreation, childbirth and a finite life span. This is roughly where Western social science theorising is at. Every book with the subtitle 'the social or cultural construction of' teases away at the fundamental distinction between cultural enterprise and natural givens. The same model can be replicated within culture. Hence one may analyse ideology as the cultural construction of other cultural values; or what one knows at one level to be an outcome of social arrangement, at another level one apprehends as a constraint. The English have always pitted against all the opportunities of an enterprising career or life-course the givens of class and childhood background, symbolised in the immutability of kin connections.

To enterprise (vb.) kinship is to touch on an area of central significance to the English − and no doubt British and European too − idea of what enterprise is all about. It collapses the idea of culture as human enterprise working against or out of nature. One will no longer think one can do nothing about the sex of one's children, about birth abnormalities and about the characteristics they will inherit, any more than one will be able to regard one's own endowment as a matter of fate. One's fate will be to put up with the results of other persons' enterprises.

There is a footnote here about the fate of a subject such as anthropology, insofar as anthropology has prided itself on its own enterprise in uncovering other people's cultures as enterprises. It uncovers what people take for granted and shows them for the cultural artefacts they are, revealing other people's naturalisms as cultural constructs. Bit of a facer, then, to find onself in a culture which is becoming cultured-up, that is, where it is not substantive products or values that are marketed but the activity of producing value itself − where what a culture values of itself is its own enterprise.

Disembodied choice

Let me end with an allegory for the reproduction of choice without body, of a culture that is all enterprise. It comes from a suggestion promoted by Howard (1988). His idea is that anthropologists, as the writers of ethnographies and the analysers of societies, should take advantage of new technology already available. The offspring of this new technology would be the hypertext.

Hypertext is produced by hypermedia − multimedia computer programming that 'allows a user to use a variety of pathways through nested information', such that a reader of hypertext 'is constantly presented with branches of information to explore and must make a series of choices while [so] exploring' (1988: 305). Hypertext is designed to be read on a screen interactively − a prospect that quite carries the author away. He imagines an ethnographic account of a wedding:

> Let me take a hypothetical example. A reader/viewer might be presented with a pictorial scene from a wedding ... One button will play a movie of the scene so that the reader can watch the ceremony performed, complete with audio. Having watched the movie, one could then examine the event as a series of stills, and explore the information nested under [a bank of] buttons. Clicking on a button attached to a person would bring up to the screen a set of new buttons, each labeled according to the kinds of information nested beneath it. One button might bring up the individual's genealogy, with information about how she is related to the bride and groom ... Another button might bring up a short biography, sketching her personal history. Within this sketch might be additional buttons leading to more detailed information, about specific roles this person plays, her achievements, responses to psychological tests, etc. Still another button might bring up a written text of things the person said during the ceremony; by clicking on specific words in the text a dictionary entry might be activated, or another button might bring up an exegesis illuminating the significance of a phrase, or other aspects of word usage. Yet another button might present an inventory of the contributions in materials and labor the person made to the event, with each item connecting to information about the nature of the items.
>
> (1988: 306−7)

The parallels with the social world of the Enterprise Culture are evident.

First, all the information is on a par. Although clumps of it are nested, one can apparently make pathways anywhere. Second, it makes evident that it is not relationships internal to the material that are being exposed, but the activity of the connecting mind that pushes the button that makes the pathways that makes the connections. Third, the apparent choice is an illusion, for two reasons. (a) The reader *has* to push the button; he or she can only make a choice. You cannot spill coffee on this text, or glance back at an earlier chapter, or suspend judgement, or just let it wash over you: you have to interact with the thing. (b) The choices are someone else's, the author's prior pathways; because the author has selected and nested the information, the reader's choices are made against the background of the author's prior ones. Nonetheless Howard (1988: 309) presents as a further 'choice' the ability of the reader to decide whether to explore information according to his/her own interests or to be guided through pre-structured pathways.

However, this last instruction throws up an assumption written into the vision of hypertext that makes it fall short of complete enterprise. It rather quaintly takes for granted that the information about the wedding exists as an extraneous datum, that is, as the body of data *about which* writer and reader are so enterprising. It is this given that allows the writer to have a creative time getting to work on the analysis of the wedding, while to the reader the nests and selections are a further given datum, and he or she has a creative time finding his or her own pathways through the information.

> The media would permit multiple relationships between textual materials and interpretation, and since so much more textual material could be included, there would be less reason to be selective ... A much wider range of materials could be accommodated, including those that did not particularly interest the ethnographer but might be of central concern to some readers.
>   (1988:307)

All the materials in the world!

One's mind reels at the possibilities. Until, of course, one realises what enterprise really means. If there is nothing that is not created by choice, one has to take away the given status of the materials themselves. Take away the independence of the background against which the choices are made. Suppose the wedding were organised *for* the multimedia.

If the couple have any cultural finesse they will be making their own hypertext. Not an album of photographs, but a computer programme in which they will be able to relive various pathways through their wedding day, depending on the preference of the moment. In fact, they may well plan the occasion with multiple interpretations in mind, think about the alternatives they will be able to present later to themselves, in short, make choices on their wedding day that they can relive as choices when they push the programme buttons. One's own pre-selected selections? Not much enterprise left for the future after all.

My account is intended as an exercise in cultural caricature — drawing attention to features through exaggeration. By the same token, the very idea of enterprise comes to seem a caricature of individual endeavour. The Enterprise Culture may well find it has not reproduced enterprise. The chances are that a culture that *thinks* itself enterprising will simply reproduce more and more technologies for its marketable reproduction.

CHAPTER 3

Future kinship
and the study of culture

On the eve of the last quarter of this century, a British volume devoted to *The Future of the Cities* (Blowers *et al.* 1974) included a speculation on 'Life in the Year 2000'. It projects a future culture. The vision of a standard of living increased four times over seems in retrospect sheer hallucination, as does the idea of a global agreement to equalise income or of custom-built submersibles for vacations in undersea resorts. But the final paragraph that deals with the health of the individual could be reprinted today without much of a blush. It also strikes the only negative note in an otherwise bright-voiced piece.

> Artificial cyborg limbs and sensory organs will be freely available; and natural transplants and synthetic implants will be commonplace. More effective contraception will be practised; and extra-uterine gestation may be chosen by some. Genetic engineering will have begun to eliminate known hereditary defects. The sex of an unborn child may be chosen ... Some of the possible developments listed above may cause us to question the basic notion of individual personality; some raise the matter of medical ethics; some would require a definite revision of social attitudes for their implementation. All we know is that they are probably going to become technologically possible. And socially, too?
>
> (Leicester 1974: 309)

* * *

The English-language concept of culture as the artefacts and artifice of, and thus created by, human enterprise developed in Britain at the time of the industrial revolution. Concepts do not exist in isolation. I describe a concatenation of ideas that have since extended the connection between artifice and creativity and others that have come to challenge it. In thinking about possible cultures for the future we might also think about whether or not this particular concept of culture will have a future.

In industrial society,* human enterprise was seen to work against the givens of the natural world. At the same time, enterprise was held to evince the very creativity that was distinctive to human nature. To call something 'artificial' carried a double meaning, conveying at once this intrinsic sense of human ingenuity and the further sense that human ingenuity could extent beyond the natural limits of human nature itself.

The artificial referred, then, to more than the adornment of humankind's natural state. Indeed it came to carry connotations derived from its latter-day creation through planned production. For the planning now required in manufacture transformed the meaning of 'industry' from that of personal effort to that of the organised utilisation of labour in a central production process. The centralisation of productive work in turn lent new resonance to other centres of human creativity such as the city. Although factories were also built in the countryside, and although industrialisation meant that places of manufacture came to be segregated from residence (Davidoff and Hall 1987), towns and cities became associated in popular thinking with industrialisation. If the town were artificial, it was not simply for the parade of manners or displays of the arts, but because its planning, time-keeping and functioning took on factory-like tenor. In Europe, Britain led the way in municipal control over public services such as gas and electricity (Rabinow 1989: 203). Speaking of French ideas at the turn of the century, Rabinow (1989: 210) writes: 'What nature and history had produced, man could bring to perfection'. And what represented that process in 'visible, palpable, bounded form' was urbanism.

Such an association between the urban and the industrial extended an older one: for Europeans the city had long represented the epitome of artifice in human life. In 1973 Williams drew attention to the almost-as-long-lived fantasy, cities of the future: 'Glittering cities have been imagined, on a thousand planets, with every kind of technical wonder' (1985: 276). Future countrysides have also been imagined, evolved beyond urban epochs where artifice no longer intrudes. Yet in the 1990s the visions of only twenty years ago seems irretrievably locked into the past. Whether the projections were of

---

* That is, before the Enterprise Culture (see Chapter 2).

megalopoloi or of de-citified 'urban fields', a creative future was projected against a stable natural environment (e.g. Blower *et al.* 1974).

We look back on the centralisation of industrial process and city life from the vantage point of one perspective. In the late twentieth century, Europeans (and their North American counterparts) can talk of de-industrialisation and de-urbanisation in the same breath. On the one hand, what appears to take the place of industry is technology. Technology in turn takes on a new character. Where industry produced, technology enables; where industry recalled the same autonomous organisation to be found in the functioning urban centre, technology carries the connotations of service. Meanwhile, 'service industry' exists as a kind of hybrid, rather less persuasive than the 'manufacturing industry' which still evokes nostalgia for the real thing (di Leonardo 1985: 254). On the other hand emerges suburbia, a kind of domestic counterpart to technology. Miyaji (in press) emphasises that among the futures projected for us lie relationships conceived as de-urbanised networks facilitated through a communications technology that can be run as well from the suburban house as from the city centre.

It might seem obvious that urbanisation should have once trailed a concatenation of ideas associated with industrialisation, organisation, the centralisation of living spaces, and so forth. What may seem less obvious is what has followed. For it means that the contemporary folk model of de-industrialisation (after di Leonardo 1985) does not present an isolated challenge. One concept is not turned on its head alone. It carries conviction precisely because it connects with others – even alliteratively in the case of de-urbanisation. The question of interest for anthropologists might well be what is happening to ideas about culture amid such devolution.

I both ask the question in a general way and explore one area of innovation – that nowadays known as reproductive technology. It is an interesting area because of the way, in Britain at least, people's attitudes mobilise the twin concepts of the artificial and the natural. Now the connection between de-urbanisation and de-industrialisation implies that those two concepts exist in mutual relationship. In the case of the contrast between the artificial and the natural, however, the effect is not of mutual reinforcement but of encroachment. The one appears to overtake or encompass the other. If childbirth was always considered a 'natural' event, late-twentieth-century advances in reproductive medicine are emphatically 'aritificial', and in a manner that outstrips the perceived artificiality of ordinary hospitalisation or medical intervention. Artifice always encroached; I shall try to show how the concept of it does too.

Perhaps a contrast between the artificial and natural will not work in Japanese in quite the way it does for English-speakers.* As we have seen, for the latter the epithet 'artificial' tends to be applied not to how people comport themselves but to what they make ('artefacts'). In the recent past, this would have meant above all one kind of artefact, namely machines. Indeed, a distinction between machine and body has for long held that between the artificial and the natural. Technology does not sustain the same distinction at all.

A concept of culture

I have introduced an emphasis of my own in the European designation of culture, that culture also consists in the way people draw analogies between different domains of their worlds. Whether as connections or contrasts, one set of ideas can always be developed to 'represent' others. Europeans regard this as itself an artificial or conventional process. I refer to 'European' to indicate the specificity of the cultural constructs under examination here, to be found in educated, middle-class circles across Northern Europe and North America.

Two observations are in order. First, if the distinction between the artificial and the natural inheres in the very idea of having a culture, it is also replicated over and again in domains themselves regarded as distinct from one another. Second, in drawing analogies, people draw attention to such (pre-existing) distinctions, and indeed in positing similarities must also posit differences. Body and machine afford an example. One basis for the distinction is that bodies have life, machines work; the one describes a natural phenomenon, the other an artificial one. However, each may in turn be used as a metaphor for the other – the body can be conceptualised as a 'machine', the machine as a 'body' (see Hayles 1990).

Throughout the twentieth century body and machine have provided parallel metaphors for the concept of culture. Europeans could think

---

* This chapter was first given to an international symposium in Japan, and before a Japanese audience.

of culture as an organic body composed of parts, even personifying it as an agent with a will and ability to act, so it was given human motivation to avoid contradiction or to impose itself on others; this was conceptualised as its natural life. Europeans were equally happy with mechanical metaphors, and could conceive of culture as a built structure with ratchet-like effects between its components; its conventions could be shown to work. These distinctions also worked at what were called different 'levels'. While at one level, a contrast between the natural and the artificial might distinguish different views of culture, it might equally distinguish Culture itself, as intrinsically artificial, from Nature, the source of all that was natural. Cultures, in this European view, were artificial creations natural to the human condition.

In the context of late-nineteenth-century industrialisation, the epoch when 'man made himself' (Wagner 1986a: 118), culture implied the acquisition of civilisation. The European study of culture attended to the evolutionary unfolding of this self-production. In the early twentieth century, anthropology underwent the metamorphosis which has given the subject its present-day shape: from the study of culture to the study of cultures (Ingold 1986). Evolutionary interest in the acquisition of civilisation was displaced by an understanding of cultures as diverse manifestations of human enterprise (Williams 1961: 18, culture as 'a whole way of life'). Each culture was conceived as being founded on its own principles and values, and thus having an independent logical status. Without this premise it is unlikely there would have been the mid-twentieth-century explosion of ethnographic, field-based studies that have since been the hallmark of anthropological enterprise. The early twenty-first century is likely to present a very different intellectual map.

The idea that cultures were autonomous meant that one could understand their life and working from the inside, as though one were dissecting an organic body or revealing the mechanism of a machine. On formal grounds they could be treated as self-contained systems. Yet almost from the start, anthropologists were taken to task for claiming their cultures were substantively isolated, unchanging and untouched. In British anthropology, this produced numerous critiques all based on the same point − that one had to consider historical process and human creativity, whether in terms of world systems or individual decision-making. On the organic analogy, metaphors of a functioning body were both extended and displaced by aetiological ones that emphasised growth and change through time. On the mechanical analogy, metaphors of structure gave way to cybernetic and topological ones producing models of information flows and processual systems. These were dominant in the 1960s and 1970s.

A similar devolution of images was already evident in society at large. The totalising impetus of British nineteenth-century factory owners, with their 'complete societies' brought under one roof (from organising every part of the working day to supervising all aspects of their workers' lives), was supplemented by a communications model of the relationships between different parts of the industrial sector. This was accompanied by an increasing compartmentalisation of people's lives through parallel civic organisations (schools, hospitals, local government offices). If the new professionalism implied in these developments gave services something of an industrial space in the early twentieth century, then in Britain these were also the decades when towns and cities began acquiring a new character in their suburbs. The town expanding against the borders of the countryside produced a new phenomenon: the semi-urban housing estate 'in' the semi-countryside.

Over the century, the growth of the service sector and the expansion of suburban living has contributed to the double sense of de-industrialisation and de-urbanisation. But while de-urbanisation is recognised in the de-centering of city amenities, the contemporary spread of suburbia has another aspect to it. It remains city-like in that it encroaches on the countryside, and thus also appears as a manifestation of creeping, global urbanisation. The late-twentieth-century world seems as much hyper-urbanised (we all have an urban identity now) as it is de-urbanised (there are no centres any more). Yet if we are all in some sense urbanised, then there is no distinctive quality to be attached to urbanisation that can be separated from life as such. There is more to this than a shift in location; we also live a conceptual shift. In retrospect, it seems that the countryside only ever seemed rural from an urban perspective. The very distinction between rural and urban has been exposed for the urban construct it is (cf. Pahl 1965). We might call this collapse of distinction a kind of suburbanisation.

Along with such a shift goes a reinterpretation of cultural change, that we live in a world simultaneously more diversified and homogenised than before. There is both 'more' culture and 'less' culture. Indeed, for the anthropologist, the spread of Western culture world-wide can seem like a de-centering process. Local identities are either hypertrophied (cultural pluralism) or atrophied (global culture is no culture). I suggest that, among things, such perceptions are an effect of what appears as encroaching artifice: now there seems nothing that is not the result of, or at least shows the encroachment of, human enterprise upon it. The point is not to be proved or disproved by measuring the quantity of enterprise: it is revealed instead in the encroachment of concepts on one another.

Metropolis and suburb

These new perceptions extend former habits of European thinking. The past tense must also be an ethnographic present insofar as the older connotations endure.

I have drawn an analogy of my own between the city as an organisation, bringing together people who have to submit to its planning as a functioning body or machine, and the model of autonomous cultures and societies that emerged in anthropological thought early in the twentieth century. The analogy is brought up to date in Hannerz's (in press) comment on the fact that the major cities of the world can be considered unique 'cultures' in their own right. But Hannerz also introduces us to other images of the city. Planning and organisation suggested artifice; this second set suggests instead what was natural to the city, namely its teeming life. Here the plenitude of persons indicated less the enhanced opportunities afforded for sociability (see Wazaki, in press) than the simple experience of diversity.

The city thus became an imaginative locus for extending the concept of culture in its own way. For the city provided a facility for the intermixing of cultural forms. The 'natural' city was a cultural marketplace, an amalgam of negotiable values, as in the 'world of the city [contained in] ... the vast flea market of Paris, where one could rediscover the artifacts of culture, scrambled and rearranged' (Clifford 1988: 121). In encapsulating the world, it was itself a cosmos. Cities thus manifested world culture; the metropolis was naturally cosmopolitan. In Hannerz's phrase, cosmopolitanism today entails an involvement with a plurality of cultures on their own terms.

Cosmopolitanism thus drew on the possibility of capturing the world in a microcosm. It might be located in the person of the individual who literally constructed a life of travel and might also be located in the way the city drew travellers to itself. It became the perpetual locus of diversity. To qualify as a city in the popular mind there had to be a cross-section of institutional enterprises (the church, the arts, commerce, government), and national divisions (class, age, occupation) as well as international ones (even if only in the collection of the world's eating places). What was 'artificial' about the city was that it encompassed cultural representatives who were regarded as torn out of context insofar as their natural origins lay elsewhere. The city thus gained its excitement from juxtapositions that were unnatural; diversity was sustained by the continued promotion of styles from distinctive sources. What appeared 'natural' were the communications and interchanges, the meeting of differences, like meetings between persons.

Culture was also imagined as a kind of person itself. This invited the thought of what happens when one culture 'met' another: the picture of culture contact. But here interchange was often imagined as one-way traffic – from the gloomy prognostications of the early twentieth century that foreign cultures were merely survivals of such encounters to the mid-century concern with colonisation as though it were a matter of one culture imposing its will upon another. Where encroachment seemed to be two-way, then the weak metaphor of a meeting was often replaced by the stronger metaphor of interbreeding. The resultant mixing of cultures could be likened to the intermarrying of different races.

Whereas the cosmopolitan who experienced the diversity of life presented an 'artificial' figure, the creole was a 'natural' embodiment of diversity in the langue he/she spoke. Creolisation is also a concept that Hannerz (1988) has applied to culture. The image of creolisation had come from the rural Caribbean, where all race was mixed race, all language the product of the coalescences and reinventions of others. To think of cultures as creolised was to think of a kind of *lingua franca* that was also a local dialect, of the way that the same transcultural elements were to be found everywhere yet at each individual place recombined in quite novel patterns. Insofar as the outcome of miscegenation was the reproduction of an entity that resembled neither of its parents, this suggested a naturally regenerative process. The new cultural body could be imagined as a unique hybrid.

Novel combinations enabled the unexpected to happen; what emerged would have a life of its own.

Cosmopolitanism has an exaggerated profile in late-twentieth-century perceptions of cities and cultures. Indeed it may subsume creolisation or hybridisation as a condition of cultural life. That life is envisaged as a process productive of unforeseen and thus hopeful outcomes. If we think of present-day cultures as the 'offspring' of past ones, we see new combinations forever being put together out of old cultural elements. Indeed, as the century has progressed, the idea has taken a hold over anthropological approaches to culture in the argument that it is not just present-day cultural forms that are cultural hybrids but that all cultures everywhere have been so. Clifford (1988) deploys it to refer to the possibility of inventive 'intercultures'.

Suspending possible differences between North America and Europe (Rapport n.d.), I note the way that Clifford transplants the term into a seemingly urban context: 'More and more people "dwell" with the help of mass transit, automobiles, airplanes. In cities on six continents foreign populations have come to stay – mixing in but often in partial, specific patterns' (1988: 13). What may have always been true of cultural mixing becomes hypertrophied in the late twentieth century. But the city is no longer the natural facilitator. In truth, this latter-day vision of an intercultural future is a suburban image, Clifford's cosmopolitans inhabiting the never-never land of transit lounges, artifice no longer contained within the bounded city but envisaged as a diffuse condition of life. Perhaps some of the current late-twentieth-century interest in intercultures, cultural hybrids or whatever does indeed come from imagining not the city but suburbia. Yet what suburbia 'represents' is highly problematic. As di Leonardo (1985: 224) shows for the idea of non-manufacturing industries in America, the very concept of the suburb seems a parasitic one.

Suburbia is neither urban nor rural. It may represent both; but when it is reproduced *as* suburbia comes to represent neither. Rather it is evidence of the encroachment of these concepts on one another. The rural, and thus the distinction between urban and rural, is re-created as a figment of the urban imagination; not as a mix of forms but as the absorption of the distinction between them. Disneyland, observes Yoshimoto (1989), does not represent America, it simulates it. It produces the imaginary distinction between the real and the imaginary. And Disneyland transported from Los Angeles to Tokyo, in turn, is neither imitation nor reproduction but an original – a real, simulated Disneyland. In the Tokyo Disneyland, he says, the distinction between the real and imaginary is exposed and thus revealed for the imaginary construction it is. Or, he might have said, between the natural and the artificial.

Continuity and change

Although it is I, as Malinowski in turn might have said, who have brought them together, these analogies for the creation of culture belong(ed) to a set of connections that an English-speaker would probably recognise. I now add a less familiar set from ideas about the creation of kinship. They provide a further dimension to the relationship between what is natural and what is artificial about the world.

This dimension concerns the European anthropologist's understanding of culture in relation to the lives of individual persons. Set against nature, culture evoked a relationship between given constraints and individual autonomy, between shared meanings and personal interpretations. This was a central preoccupation of mid-twentieth-century anthropology. In the way these concepts were played off against each other (cf. Parkin 1987) we can also see between them an oscillation between focusing on what is fixed or immutable in social life and what is open to change and innovation. A sense of change was seen against a sense of constraint, future possibility against what was assumed to be given. This interplay was characteristic both of the way anthropological models of culture developed over the last few decades, and also of middle-class folk models of the nature of human relations evinced in their constructions of kinship.

As in the case of the distinction between the natural and the artificial, this contrast operated at different 'levels'. Thus kinship as a whole could be represented as a (natural) domain based on immutable relations as against the rest of society; or, in the way that kin arranged their relationships, we might discern within the domain of kinship both what could not be changed (a natural element) and what could be (an artificial one). The English could draw on the family as a metaphor for thinking about continuity and change alike. For families might either appear as autonomous entities with their own traditions, as constellations of unique properties (and property) transmitted between generations, based on a line of natural ancestry; or they might appear as constellations of individuals who worked together or who moved away from one another, and who in any case diversified their interests, renegotiated their obligations and chose with whom they associated. Indeed, these two images of the family formed a pair: the relationships given by immutable blood ties were set against the potential mobility of individual members. The one image both covered and revealed the other. For what was not open to change (the given ties of blood) could be either valued or ignored in the choice people had to conduct their own lives. Thus the individual interpreted for him-/herself the claims of 'tradition'. This was very similar to the conventional mid-century anthropological understanding of culture as a traditional body of 'shared' values and attitudes that individuals constantly reinterpreted or realised or challenged in their own lives.

If this latter view of culture is becoming increasingly hard to sustain (cf. Cohen's critique, 1987), should we be drawing instead on the idea of the cosmopolitanised and always plural culture, or even perhaps the creolised language? Despite the apparently exotic origins of these constructs, they too resonate with English ideas about procreation. There was a sense in which all breeding was miscegenation and all offspring hybrids. The sense was, of course, a metaphoric one.

Children were, in the English view, genetic hybrids by nature: they were regarded as constellations of elements derived from each parent but mixed in such a way as to make them into unique entities with a future that repeated the past of neither mother nor father. The uniqueness of the person as an individual was thus replicated in the supposed genetic constitution. Moreover, this spontaneous hybridisation has, in the recent past, been regarded as a source of hope for the future – it is what made every generation of children 'new' children. An important factor was the element of chance built into the process. One knew what the parents were like but could only make partial predictions from them about the children. Between parents and children, parents were fixed, immutable points of reference, children unpredictable, their future lying ahead. What the latter would be like depended in part on the chance outcome of the moment of conception. Out of human control, that lay with nature.

At the same time, the sheer multiplication of the generations meant that with the passage of time there were more persons who had lived in the world and more evidence of human enterprise upon it. The sphere of human control was thought to be continually expanding. Just as the city seemed to be a source of cultural change, so it seemed natural for the artificial to encroach upon the natural, a kind of covert evolutionism that assumed the future would be characterised by more change not less, by cultures increasingly rather than decreasingly creolised, by tradition becoming fainter. Out of this set of ideas has come the late-twentieth-century perception of an ever more crowded human population on the earth, and of the natural world as more than ever subject to artificial management, or accident for that matter: there seems nothing now that is not amenable to legislation, protection and conservation, or prey to exploitation and bungling. What is 'given' shrinks under the onslaught of what human beings can 'create'. Nature becomes a department of human enterprise, and we discover that it was never autonomous. The distinction between the natural and the cultural is revealed for the cultural construction it always was.

The natural world, including the facts of human biology, is in the late twentieth century no longer taken for granted. However culture is redefined, its distinctive characteristic as human enterprise working against the givens of nature seems already to belong to the past. As far as the interests of anthropologists are concerned, recent issues in the conceptualisation of kinship will certainly affect the future way in which one is to think about the relationship between what is given and what is open to human enterprise, and thus of the ambiguous connection between creativity and artifice. The issues are quite overtly spoken of as artificial intervention in a supremely natural process. They also comprise a phenomenon that belongs definitively to the last quarter of the twentieth century.

Natural and artificial procreation

On the face of it, nothing today seems further from erosion than the concept of nature. Against a background of concern about the natural environment, constant reference is made to what is also natural in human behaviour, and nowhere is it more emphasised than in the debates over the new reproductive technologies. (Recent academic collections include Stanworth (1987); Spallone and Steinberg (1987), in the wake of the Report of the Committee of Inquiry into Human Fertilisation and Embryology established in 1982 (Warnock 1985);

the Glover Report on Reproductive Technologies to the European Commission appeared in 1989.) Here technology appears not as a service to industrial production, making machines work (see Ingold, 1988), but as a service to human reproduction, making bodies live. In its benign aspect, it enables people to fulfil their desires.

These particular technologies thus intervene in the very area that has in the past provided Europeans with analogies for the vigorous hybrid creativity of the future − whether on the unique individual or the born-again culture − namely human procreation. Human beings were regarded as naturally fertile, and the acts of procreation were normally regarded as natural acts. Today, if couples 'fail' to have children by such methods, then it is becoming increasingly possible for them to seek assistance. A medical booklet put out by Serono Laboratories (UK) Ltd, to advertise drugs for the stimulation of ovulation, has the title 'If nature can't deliver'. It may be the gametes themselves, or the process of fertilisation or of implantation in the womb that has to be supplemented. Consequently, the intervention − artificial insemination by donor, egg donation, *in vitro* fertilisation (IVF), maternal surrogacy − is of a remedial nature. Such intervention is 'artificial', but far from creating an autonomous domain of enterprise (as in industrial production), it is presented as directly responsive to fundamental natural process. Its power is bio-power, replicating the (ideal) potencies of the body (Braidotti 1988). There is always *some* portion of the reproductive process that is marked as demonstrably natural.

Thus IVF may enable the natural parents to have children of their own genetic endowment; or the gamete material of one or other parent may be supplemented by that of another person but brought to term by the mother-to-be, and so forth. At its most evident, what remains as the natural element may simply be the desire to have children by some form of childbirth as distinct from adoption. Assisting conception thus emerges as the most prominent target of medical research, of the setting up of clinics, and of public interest.

As long as some element of the entire process of childbirth can be claimed as 'natural', technological intervention appears enabling. But I suggest there is a subtle shift from regarding naturalness as part of the workings of physiology to attributing it to parental desire. On the one hand, desire becomes translated into the choice whether or not to adopt certain procedures, and choice is thereby exercised as choice between different artificial possibilities; in this sense it is limited. But, on the other hand, as a natural dimension to human creativity, desire itself is supposedly without limits.

Two versions of a booklet prepared by Organon, a research-oriented pharmaceutical company, lay the groundwork. The booklet is designed to allay fears about IVF. Both versions assert that a natural element remains in the process. One puts it thus:

> *You have a natural desire* for children and may have been trying for some time without success. Don't despair, there is still hope; thanks to major advances in medical science, many couples who were previously considered infertile can now produce healthy babies.

The second:

> This booklet focuses attention upon one technique, in particular, in vitro fertilization (fertilization that takes place outside the human body). It must be stressed that although fertilization occurs outside the body, the development and formation of a child takes place, *naturally, inside the womb.*

The one stresses the naturalness of the womb, the other the naturalness of parental desire. Desire appears as natural as the womb. In either case, both state the nature of the assistance: 'Nature sometimes needs a helping hand'.

Nature assisted compromises the definition of nature as those conditions of life from which intervention is absent; what is given is no longer given by nature itself but is visibly circumscribed by technological capability. That in turn will force certain choices on people in the future. (In 1987 it was reported that some 3000 frozen embryos were stored in Britain ('stockpiled', *Guardian* 5.10.87), perhaps 10,000 world-wide; two years later the figure suggested for Europe alone is 20,000 (*Wall Street Journal* 26.9.89). Decisions have to be taken on their future life.) At the same time, the enabling capacity of technology appears to give it a further sinister edge. Questions are raised about the moral or ethical status of the desires it enables people to realise. Thus does 'assisting nature' slide into 'assisting human desire'. The *Sunday Express* (2.11.89, paragraphing ignored) published an alarmist story on the lack of regulation in access to AID:

> Single women who want to have babies without the emotional ties of a husband are using artificial insemination clinics in growing numbers. The revelation comes amid growing alarm over the lack of legislative

control covering Britain's rapidly increasing donor sperm business. The British Pregnancy Advisory Service, which has insemination clinics around the country, reports a 'remarkable and still escalating' number of women coming to them who are unmarried and not in a stable relationship.

Quite clearly the newspaper felt that the choices being made by these unmarried women should involve public adjudication; not all desires should be assisted.

Whether positively or negatively, the new technology is seen as enlarging the spheres open to human choice: procedures of sex selection are intended to help couples at risk of giving birth to children with sex-linked diseases; embryonic removal and inspection is done with the intention that only healthy embryos will be reimplanted, and so forth. These particular examples come from newspaper reports (*Today* 7.9.89 and *Observer* 24.1.88), for such technological developments are an endless source of more or less sensational copy.

And the sensationalism comes from the future orientation of the debate (cf. Lowenthal 1990). The fear that the Organon booklet tries to allay is an anticipatory emotion. Wilson refers to the pervasive future orientation of research on home technology and networking, 'assessed, analyzed, and written about in anticipation of its future introduction' (1988: 3), but he is wrong in supposing it has few parallels. Speculation on the future of reproductive practices is in the same position and there are similar results. Such studies cannot attend to the 'specific economic, political and social conditions as a way of interpreting their meaning for society' (1988: 3–4), for these conditions also lie in the future. The result is that the parameters of the technology seem self-determining. An ideological consensus, in Wilson's terms, is created in terms of the technological potential, which is then seen simply as human potential. Those who do not see the potential do not understand that technology can make life work! The opposing view, that the new reproductive technologies are failed technologies, has a struggle to find a voice (e.g. Klein 1989). That is partly because of the current connotations of technology. Insofar as they are enabling, medical practices perceived as technologies assist persons to realise their desires. They cannot 'fail' to assist, even where the desire itself is not in the end realised.

What is taken for granted is that technology is about the future. 'Children of the Future' is the headline to the *Daily Mail*'s (2.10.87) reporting of one of the first cases of surrogacy following *in vitro* fertilisation. Technological encroachment is exactly what twentieth-century Europeans see as the future. Hence the readiness to project; what is projected are the kinds of choices that might be made possible by the new technologies. Thus people may talk in the same breath of cloning as they do of IVF, and there are fears that 'scientists' will promote certain procedures simply in order to produce human genetic material on which they can experiment. Indeed, an editorial in the *New Scientist* (3.12.87), reporting on the first appearance of the White Paper *Human Fertilisation and Embryology* (HMSO 1987), regretted that the Paper regarded it necessary to propose 'an outright ban on research aimed at creating human clones, ape–human hybrids or genetically engineered babies'. The White Paper, the editorial argued, had done irreparable damage by its futurist projection, depriving itself of its own regulative intent in evoking the damaging image of maverick scientists interested in borderline research. They noted that all the national newspapers but one began their report on the White Paper with the ban on cloning. But, then, an article in the *Wall Street Journal* (26.9.89) commenting on the award of custody of seven frozen embryos in a Tennessee court to their 'biological mother' (against the wishes of her ex-husband), concluded with the following paragraph:

> Science and technology have far outpaced the law and traditional ethics. There are even more stunning prospects for the future: cloning; growing human embryos in the laboratory as a source of organs for transplant surgery; women giving birth to their own brothers and sisters or grand-children; widespread womb-leasing and surrogacy; animal–human and human–robot hybrids; the use of artificial, animal or dead women's wombs to incubate human embryos; and genetic engineering.

Yet for the student of culture, the point is surely that law and traditional ethics will never catch up. If there are seemingly no barriers to what is open to artificial intervention, then there are seemingly no givens either, and nowhere else for law and traditional ethics to exist. Certainly, we cannot rely on nature to impose its own limits. The principal reason, I suggest, is the manner in which we reveal to ourselves the fact that we see we cannot rely on human nature.

Europeans in the late twentieth century know that *they* do not want human–animal hybrids, that spare-parts surgery should be kept within medical limits, and that if it is no real confusion of kin relations to have sisters donate eggs to one another, there is certainly something awry about mother–daughter substitutions. But they cannot count on future generations not wishing for these things. The prospects of future enterprise leads to as much fear as hope – not that the artificial might be less than the real thing, but for the real things it might in fact make. Artifice: new choices are opened up, new possibilities for the realisation of human desires. Creativity: new possibilities create desires that from our present vantage point do not seem human at all.

For the European anthropologist, the concept of culture is already problematised. It is not at all clear what is or is not an artefact. The point is not that the boundaries between bodies and machines are theoretically troublesome (Ingold 1988; Hayles 1990), but that we now live in a world that makes explicit to itself the *ability* to breach the difference. The NRT are but one area where the body (that lives) and the machine (that works) are imagined in new conjunctions.

This particular pair (body, machine) were formerly connected and contrasted by analogy, in that they provided metaphors for different aspects of human nature. It is their metaphorical status that now seems subject to encroachment. Technology literally helps 'life' to 'work'. No doubt people will go on talking about assisting nature in the same way as they talk of releasing engineered life-forms 'into' an environment that they have already altered. Yet insofar as they cannot evoke distinctive domains of life, bodies and machines can no longer serve as metaphors for one another. It follows that the relation between them will become a poor analogy for contrasting what is given in the world with what is artificial, the basis upon which the anthropological concept of culture has rested throughout the twentieth century. It is not the challenge to the substantive concept that must be of most interest to anthropology, but the challenge to the conventional facility to draw analogies.

* * *

Whatever is said about the blurring of the idea of the city, about being unable to pin down an identity that is urban or post-urban, hyper-urban or de-urbanised, or whatever is said about the miscegenation of cultures turning into replications of the same differences, I suspect that such conceptions also constitute a response to other shifts in the conceptualisation of human relationships. Technological innovation invites us to think innovatively about how persons are born and the relatives they are born to. Yet instead of the potential of unexpected combinations, the creation of unique individuals and unplanned effects, the future seems increasingly trapped by present choice. It is as though creativity were trapped by artifice. Europeans can look to future kinship to provide them neither with metaphors for the natural givens of human existence nor with metaphors for regeneration through the spontaneous effects of procreation.

PART II

Chapter 4   'Between a Melanesianist and a Deconstructive Feminist' was the full title of this article published by *Australian Feminist Studies*, and written in 1988 in response to Vicki Kirby

Chapter 5   'Parts and Wholes: Refiguring Relationships in a Postplural World' formed a contribution to Adam Kuper's panel, 'Conceptualising Societies', at the inaugural meeting of the European Association of Social Anthropologists, Coimbra, 1990

CHAPTER 4

Between a Melanesianist and a feminist

From within the impossible space of an 'inbetween' theory and practice, that space in which women ... live out the paradox of their existence, can a specifically feminist critique gather its peculiar energies.

(Kirby 1989: 7)

On one issue several scholarly practices of the 1980s seem agreed: to make a deliberate contrivance out of undoing the assumptions that formerly held disciplines in place. That includes undoing their modes of discourse. The converse is that attention to language (as a vehicle for discourse) will expose the very practice of construction as such. In its evident capacity to be taken apart, language has thus acquired something of a special status, as though all words composed texts, as though all forms were literary forms. For any literary form can be exposed as rhetoric; any text can be made to show its plot, its structure, the claims that underpin its authority.

No surprise that feminist scholarship should have anticipated this mood. With no single discipline to defend – though produced within many – it has indeed deliberately contrived to slip between (Kirby 1989: 11), and it would be comforting to think of this paper as an attempt to live between discourses, feminist and anthropological, a new authority that is not an authority. On the other hand, if deconstruction is 'self-confessedly parasitic upon the metaphysical discourses it is out to subvert' (Moi 1985: 39), then perhaps the same is true of feminist scholarship – in which circumstances one might prefer to be parasite than host. But not everything is open to preference. I am brought up against the possibility that differences negotiable from one perspective appear non-negotiable from any other. As an anthropologist I remain committed to the interesting idea that there are vocabularies that exceed the most contrived excesses of the language in which Western scholars write (cf. Moore 1988), and as a Melanesianist I encounter a positioning of the sexes that makes their isomorphism as significant as their difference. Nonetheless, as always, my comment on certain feminist positions is equally a comment on certain social science ones. Perhaps the sense of debt I feel towards feminist scholarship indicates my sometimes parasitism upon it.*

Incomplete culture

To anthropologists used to thinking of culture as a text, the discovery that texts are cultural productions has made instant sense. Accounts appear 'constructed' in the way that cultures are.[1] The text that purports to be about (another) culture is indeed a 'text', a cultural artefact from its own.

But what *kind* of text? There seems a common assumption that once anthropologists are aware of the texted nature of writing, they will know how to deal with it. Prescriptions about dialogue and heteroglossia go hand in hand with a critical practice that uncovers the layering of narrative, a dismantling that implies that all texts are put together in the same way: susceptible to multiple reading, containing traces of other texts, partial utterances that evoke what has not been said. Certainly, that is how 'cultures' and 'societies' seem put together. Indeed, the notion of a construction that is itself partial, like a collage that never entirely suppresses the alterity of its composite elements, has become an anthropological enthusiasm of the 1980s. A potent example is the cultural/social construction of the body.[2] Again, the assumption seems to be that once we are aware of artifice in the way the body is presented we shall know how to deal with it analytically, a point which feminist interests have shown is rather more difficult than might be imagined. Artifice can be demonstrated, however, precisely because it seems partial; like a text replete with ruptures, gaps, elisions, it never completely 'describes' the body.

One source of cultural or social constructionist[3] theorising is Berger's and Luckman's work; I quote from a recent rendition:

> Berger (1967) sees the infant as incomplete, it cannot become human outside of society and its dependent and partially formed human nature at birth necessitate(s) a lengthy primary socialisation. During this period

---

* The essay incurred debts of its own, in particular to Lisette Josephides, Andrew Lattas and James Weiner for their comments, and to Susan Magarey.

the child inherits culture and language as natural objects in the world.
Most children become linguistically competent in their natal language
which ... depicts and interprets their experience. The self is received and
complementary to language. It is only at a later stage of socialisation
that the possibility of alternative worlds and thus an alternative self [is]
realised.

(Yates 1988: 14)

Culture in this formula stands equally for society. The clinching
analogy is that culture and language are alike learned, versions of
reality imposed on the learning child. Persons reach further understandings of themselves from the culture or language itself, insofar
as to reflect on the received forms is to expose the possibility of
alternatives.

Yet the concreteness of the image – the learning child – also
gives pause for thought. Suppose another image is put in its place
(J. Weiner 1988: 9), drawn from the real-life imaginings of people,
in this case Melanesians. Suppose the infant person is not regarded
as incomplete; suppose there is nothing to construct?

The power of the aesthetic analogy between cultures and texts is
also the limitation of its imagery. Cultures/societies – like persons –
are perceived as composed, and forever in the process of being so.
For scholars who have to compose their accounts, this may be an
inevitable perception. Yet we have to take pains that it does not completely conceal situations where people act on the basis of different
perceptions.

Such differences are not to be elicited naively from the actor's
viewpoint. They can exist only as an outcome of theoretical work
(Rabinow 1988), elicited from previous theoretical positions. An
example is the underpinning of the constructionist thesis by the concept of socialisation. The 'need' to transmit and pass on culture,
much as property is passed on, is presented as a general human condition, and a precondition for continuity. It seems so obvious that
children have to 'learn' culture, 'learn' social rules, just as they
learn a language, it is assumed other peoples perceive the same need.
Anthropologists may thus take practices such as initiation rites as
deliberate instruments of socialisation. The actors' intention is read
as a desire to make children into adults by equipping them with the
appropriate apparatus, by moulding them into shape.

Initiation rites hold our attention, I suspect, because of their focus
on the body. As the medium through which the initiands receive the

imprint of culture, mutilated or forced into unnatural positions, the body presents a vivid image of 'construction'. We appear to be literally witnessing the formation of the cultural or social person, and the passage from childhood to adulthood becomes a metonym for all the processes by which persons are so moulded.

Socialisation could thus be said to mimic the manner in which persons are forced into a mould that does not take their authentic form. Insofar as this other form is perceived, it provides grounds for resistance. Authenticity is often symbolised as a private or essential aspect of the person. For Westerners reflect on the way natural or biological process submits to human intervention, as when Tabet argues that reproduction is no spontaneous manifestation of the female body. Between the capacity to procreate and the fact of birth lies the relationship between the sexes, and the history of relations of reproduction, a history 'in large part of reproduction as exploitation' (Tabet 1987: 3). Indeed, her analysis of the technical control of processes such as giving birth resonates with Martin's more general findings about American women's perceptions. Childbirth is part of women's lifelong experience of managing their bodies in resistance to prevalent forms of thought that would impose certain regimens of time and behaviour. She writes:

> numerous contrasts dominate postindustrial capitalist society: home versus work, sex versus money, love versus contract, women versus men. Because of the nature of their bodies, women far more than men cannot help but confound these distinctions every day. For the majority of women, menstruation, pregnancy, and menopause cannot any longer be kept at home. Women interpenetrate what were never really separate realms. They literally embody the opposition, or contradiction, between the worlds.
>
> (1987: 197)

The women in her study felt they were carried along 'by forces beyond their control' (1987: 12); for they had a vantage point from which to see those forces as apart from themselves.

> In a multitude of ways women assert an alternative view of their bodies, react against their accustomed social roles, reject denigrating scientific models, and in general struggle to achieve dignity and autonomy ...
>
> Because their bodily processes go with them everywhere, forcing them to juxtapose biology and culture, women glimpse every day a conception of another sort of social order. At the very least, since they do not fit into the ideal division of things (private, bodily processes belong at home),

they are likely to see that the dominant ideology is partial: it does not capture their experience.

(1987: 400)

Women, she suggests, derive their sense of experience from a body that is not completely encompassed by these cultural categories. In this regard, it is not the person but the culture which is incomplete.[4]

But is a completed culture, or society, conceivable? If so, surely it would not be *perceived* as in the process of construction. Concomitantly, if people did not regard one another as having to learn culture the way language is learned, perhaps they would not apprehend their social practices as compositions. In that case, they would have no interest in the images we find so compelling. If discourse is not imagined as a text or performances as scripted, then presumably there would be no problem about the relationship of the plot to the character or the plan to the model or the model to the structure, or of lived experience to cultural category. There would be no conern with how to assemble raw materials, to make a whole out of parts, to make individuals aware of society. And perhaps there would not be the same preoccupation with the partial nature of representation.

The present wave of criticism in anthropology is much preoccupied with the relationship between what is said and not said, with giving inaudible actors a voice, with looking between lines at the interstices. The process may be visualised as discovering a space. To conceive of what is made visible as space, or to conceive of space as absence, comes of course from a prior concept of language or culture as a set of positive but partial relationships between 'things'. Thus Martin's American women are able to 'see the inextricable way our cultural categories are related and to see the falseness of the dichotomies' (Martin 1987: 200). In this view, to think of what is left unsaid can come upon one as a realisation of another dimension. The power is of imagining absence as a kind of presence, as in recalling other authors whose authority the anthropologiest displaces, or making present the 'absence' of the perceptible body whose functions have no ostensible presence in social/cultural practices.

Yet people who do not regard culture as constructed, as sets of relations between things, would not have 'our' interest in *discovering* such spaces. On the contrary, we may find that they deliberately create absences, deliberately erase the memory of events,[5] create relations not by bringing persons together but by separating them,[6] and far from being troubled by what is unsaid, make it part of everyday discourse on discourse that words are elusive. Such at least is commonly reported from Melanesia.[7] Indeed, Melanesians may assume that words are deceptive. Language is too light to carry the weight of learning and structuring with which Westerners sometimes invest it. Certainly there are Melanesians who might find odd the suggestion that one could expose authority or subvert ideology through manipulating words.[8] Rather, alternative meanings, like other persons, are always present.

Incomplete feminism

Whether through disinterral or through mimicry to excess, it is through word usage that recent feminist critics have attempted to subvert the pressure of phallocentric discourse (cf. Weedon 1987). Conversely, failure to destabilise one's language by means of strategies such as metaphoric overlay, ramification and elision is held to betray a commitment to the old order. This indeed is Kirby's (1989) criticism of my work (Strathern 1985a). She points out that insofar as my writing is naive of deconstructive practice, it is bogged down in the kind of binarisms by which anthropology's treatment of 'the other' is also to be criticised. I am politically contaminated without having the vision to exploit that contamination. In fact, although her critique addresses one article, it is telling in the context of other work where I purport to describe varieties of Anglophone feminist scholarship, yet where 'deconstructive feminism' is not even on the list.

I am provoked, then, to think about how deconstructive practice, or talk of it, is pressed into the service of a feminist scholarship that also deals with issues with which anthropologists deal. Kirby (1989: 20) refers to feminists as 'cultural critics'. What conceptualisation of culture leads one to argue, as she does, for the possibility of cultural disruption? It can only be, I think, the idea of culture as a construction.

> A feminism which enjoys slippery-dipping *on the between slides of a culture's meanings or margins* risks exceeding the repetition of a self-same, homogenised, controllable (b)order – an exhilarating risk that will be remarked treacherous, subversive, irrational. A feminism within anthropology can revel in the feeling that its pleasures escape the discipline's use-values, using its axioms only to make them slide and collide against each other until they weaken and begin to fracture.
> (1989: 19, my emphasis)

A coercive machine; in protest against my attachment to binarisms she writes:

> Strathern's attempt to forestall requires the forestalling of the debate itself rather than the careful deconstruction of its terms. I think it better to argue against the violent appetite of the Hegelian dialectic from the position one is *made to occupy* within it. Although trapped inside the 'mechanism', there is no better place from which to connive a disruptive interruption in its machinery.
>
> (1989: 19, my emphasis)

Moreover, whatever others may claim for the relationship between deconstruction and postmodernism,[9] she distinguishes feminism's concerns in the same way as the female body gives distinction to women's reflections.

> In spite of Postmodernism's promise of ambiguity and multiplicity, of other voices and spaces appearing in representational texts, its rhetoric often weaves an aesthetic closure against 'old narratives' which spoke of power, positions and commitments. Within contemporary 'avant-garde' discourse, the metaphor of woman operates as signifier of the labyrinth, the cryptic, the uncanny doublefold within which the excess of meaning is enclosed/hidden even as its truth is confounded in an eternal riddle. But for woman herself, she is always positioned within the corporeal significance of her material embodiment. She is placed, or 'naturalised', within the endless mutations of femininity's masquerades. These symbolic representational demands plot the real dimensions through which her life is lived, understood, and hence truly fathomed in its actual significance.
>
> (1989: 20)

Her intention is not to destroy or transcend the everyday world of meanings/values but to give them political intent:

> the necessity *which woman's body provides a space* from which a new morpho-logic for thinking and speaking can be generated, also acts to guarantee the stalling of a 'post political' slippage into postmodernism's threatened positionlessness.
>
> (1989: 20, my emphasis)

The promise is of terrorism, a continual disruption of the machinery. For while there is no suggestion that we are not all implicated in their perpetuation, language and culture are personified as having a generic male authorship.[10] One reinscribes what has been described by other interests. Only the presumption that language has indeed been manufactured to 'other' specifications could make such a movement political and subversive.

This movement can be imagined as a passage between what is on the surface and what is concealed. It is a powerful attraction of deconstructive talk that it talks about getting between, underneath or beyond words, betraying their fixity by showing how they can be dissolved into one another, unscaffolding the divide between interior and exterior. Instead of scrutinising words for their 'real' meanings, they are refracted, de-essentialised.

Such a politicised critique of logocentrism suggests culture and language can in turn be imagined as sustained to the advantage of some. To slip in between things is to reveal how partial the constructions are: meanings could only be made by some at a cost to others, and the traces of that cost and those others remain enigmatically there. Slippage 'between', as Kirby advises, recovers the unintended alterity, or the inadvertent oversight, like the omission of feminist contributions from *Writing Culture*, with respect to the otherwise determining but thereby incomplete culture.

Some of these points are recapitulated by Threadgold. She argues that the microstructure of texts acts as a 'realisation of, a metaphor for, social structure and culture' (1988: 42), such that language is only ever an aspect of context, and context is constructed of language. 'Texts are constructed of other texts, other voices, the voices of the heteroglossia of the culture and the social system' (1988: 42). However, the problem of making words mean is not an exclusively feminist one, for it is not language that men control but access to valued modes of meaning. What men and women do with language shows 'how the *doing* is constrained by *existing* power relations, subjective coding orientations, and access to genres and discourses' (1988: 64, original emphasis). In her view it is not language that oppresses but the economic, political and discursive forms which control differential access. We need

a non-hierarchical articulation of masculine and feminine in language which would not maintain it as an opposition or reverse it or equalise it but would involve the construction of alterity for men and women *in their difference* ... But it will only come about through generic change and a view of what language is which would involve the displacement/ overturning of the value-laden dichotomies which are still implicit in arguments that would see women speaking, as bodies, in intonation and fractured syntaxes and leave men (still disembodied) speaking in grammar and logic.

(1988: 65–6, original emphasis)

Deliberate contrivance is thus required to overcome reinstatement of the dichotomies against which feminists argue in promoting their counter-reality of feminine bodies.[11] Yet it is contrivance itself which produces such inadvertent endorsements of the concepts one tries to erode.[12] The alternatives appear to be between logic and its fracturing: slipping is subversive because words are otherwise significant in themselves, is liberating because language otherwise imprisons meaning.

One result, Threadgold suggests, is that Anglo-American readings are mis-matched with the new genres of French feminist texts.

> Kristeva's and Irigaray's theory of language read *literally* is involved in maintaining the very dichotomies, the logocentrism and metaphysics which they and Derrida and social semiotic theory have set out to deconstruct. *In fact* however, their theoretical practice, which uses these notions *metaphorically* is extra-ordinarily powerful. Their texts *must* be read as *metaphor, play, paradox* − and as generic subversion. Only a different genre of reading will prevent the reassertion of the metaphysics of presence through their work.
>
> (Threadgold 1988: 63, original emphasis)

For example, Alcoff (1988) sees post-structuralist feminists as attacking the concept of the oppressed authentic subject, in the double claim that there is no authentic subject and no oppression in the humanist sense. Since this makes us all 'constructs' (1988: 16), she concludes that a deconstructing feminism can only be a negative strategy, the assertion of total difference that cannot be pinned down or subjugated within a dichotomous hierarchy. 'The political struggle can only have [in Kristeva's words] "negative function", "rejecting everything finite, definite, structured, loaded with meaning, in the existing state of society" ' (Alcoff 1988: 418).

With Threadgold, we might say that Kristeva is commenting metaphorically on the impossibility of neither occupying nor not-occupying a space or position. Alcoff reads her literally as proposing an unworkable political practice. Hence, she avers, feminism needs to explore a theory of a gendered subject (an individual self or 'agent'); her solution is to comprehend woman as positioned by a network of relations. Women can 'use their positional perspective as a place from which values are interpreted and constructed rather than as a locus of an already determined set of values' (Alcoff 1988: 434). Alcoff appears content to discover women's positioning as the space they *happen* to occupy − an accidental or inadvertent location.

The significant point seems that, wherever she is, 'the identity of a woman is a product of her own interpretation and reconstruction of her history' (Alcoff 1988: 434).

Threadgold and Alcoff, linguist and philosopher, are both concerned with political practice, but where one sees verbal play as the subject's potential subversion of genres (including 'subjectivity'), the other wishes to make subjectivity itself literally visible as 'a fluid interaction in constant motion and open to alternation by self-analyzing practice' (Alcoff 1988: 425). Insofar as these examples show a diversity of approaches towards deconstructive feminism, the point is taken against myself that in the late 1980s any account of feminist scholarship is incomplete without traces of deconstructive practice.

* * *

There is a personal irony to this. Not only was my first book on Melanesia called *Women in Between*, I found myself *writing the word 'deconstruction' out of* a more recent one (1988), hesitating to appropriate a term to whose theoretical contextualising I had no access. Of course, that is being scrupulous after the event: the idea had already done its work in the text.

Yet to what idea did 'deconstruction' seem applicable? My usage was not informed by literary and philosophical subtleties. Given the overall argument that the people of Melanesia do not work with concepts of society and culture, I simply wished to upturn the familiar Western notion that society is 'constructed' by describing collective activities which apparently aim at an opposite effect. Group relations as they appear in clan engagements or initiation rituals are effective to the extent that they take pre-existing relations apart. However, the terms deconstitution and decomposition conveyed my meaning.

Without calling it thus perhaps I was nonetheless describing 'deconstructive practice'. Melanesians take relations apart by uncovering hidden layers; they bring to the surface what is not said, evoke shadow presences, allow of no final summary or gloss, and indeed act out a gender alterity of such sophistication that would make a Westerner blanch. Moreover these practices are to be found in stretches of events, in performances that have, like written texts, a specifiable aesthetic form.

But there is also a difference, and that concerns the relationship of accident and contrivance. Their inversions and juxtapositions are not perceivable as incidental oversight or the disinterral of suppressed otherness, and revelation of multiple, hidden meaning is not necessarily subversive. On the contrary, public utterances may be regarded as subversive[13] and multiple interpretations deliberately contrived. A person or artefact with one set of connotations may in the course of a performance be radically re-presented in another.[14] It is *assumed* that such deliberate action often works by bringing the interior to the surface. Indeed, this aesthetic is all-pervasive: there is no recognised form − a men's house, male and female bodies, a gift of food − that is not subject to such decomposing effort. But the 'meanings' of such acts are always the same: to make evident people's social (cultural) capability, or sociality.

When sociality is routinely elicited through successive presentations, one concrete image displaces another equally concrete image. Interpretations may be idiosyncratic, readings in that sense multiple, but the form each image itself takes is 'complete' (Wagner 1991). As far as words or the performance is concerned, there is no in-between to be brought to light. There is nothing as it were that is not either hidden *or* revealed. For what is hidden is hidden till it is revealed; and what is revealed is revealed in order to be hidden. Unlike positivist discursive practice which assumes that something brought to the surface will stay there, and unlike such deconstructionism as assumes an infinite dissemination of reference, Melanesians work at hiding again what they have made known. For they make an assumption of particularism but not essentialism. When one reveals something one does not reveal its essence or secret: one reveals that it contains something else! You cannot look inside a person to discover the true person: you will instead find other (particular) persons.

Now while the cross-disciplinary popularisation of deconstructive practice enabled me to think about Melanesia in certain ways, Melanesians' practices cannot be presented as an example *of* it. They are not doing deconstruction in the Western sense because they do not hold constructionist premises. If sociality is immanent, there can be no perceived effort to either 'construct' or 'deconstruct' it.

Yet if my problem is why I had to write deconstruction out of a work on Melanesia, conversely there may be good reason to write it in *apropos* Western society. I propose to contrive a separation between the Western and the Melanesian cases in order to capitalise on Kirby's critique of binarism, to glance at another way of conveying similarity and difference that does not require the ontology of an oppositional economy. However, it requires differentiating between means and ends.

The end is to exemplify certain dual but non-binary ways of imaging derived from my understanding of Melanesian symbolic procedures. Different forms may be perceived as substituting for one another in such a way that each entirely occupies the other's space, as an alternative that is neither the simple inverse nor negation of the prior form. Thus we might imagine adult and child, parent and offspring: what in Western binary thinking could be conceptualised as opposites, in the Melanesian formulations I wish to convey are conceptualised as unmediated recapitulations or refigurings of each other. One consequence is that there is no 'between' here, no gap or distance between the two forms. (Other ways of imagining such relations do take a mediated form, as when two parties are regarded as exchanging characteristics between them, and thus creating a relationship which is neither of them. I am not concerned with those symbolisations here.) In order to make the refigurings appear, however, Melanesians may set up dichotomies, as between interior and exterior. There is no flickering in between of interiority or exteriority, as Kirby would like, but indeed a displacement.[15] So male may be seen to contain female, and vice versa, without there being anything blurred or ambiguous about either gender. The one is a version of the other in a 'different' shape.

In order to make this other form of thinking appear one that is not the inverse or negation of Western forms, for it was not developed in relation to them, I am constrained by the fact that there is, of course, no 'Melanesian case' that is not a Western projection. I therefore deliberately 'reveal' it through a binarism firmly located in an us/them contrast that works by inversion and negation. These are my means. Not the infinite regression of third (mediating) terms, but a strategy of displacement. I thus try to present Western discourse as a form through which Melanesian discourse can appear. If one thinks about it, 'Melanesian discourse' can, of course, have no other locus. Yet the transparency of the fiction will, I hope, simultaneously indicate that the life of the one form is not pre-empted by the other, and is certainly not a residual to it.

'Conception and de-conception'

Two striking features emerged from Martin's analysis. First, women's capacity to resist social convention through their bodies and their access to absent or overlooked experiences are normally suppressed 'below the surface' of everyday life. Second, diverse physiological functions appear gathered together in Western discourse as 'a body'. Things that happen to different parts are thus regarded as taking apart the body, so that the person to whom the body belongs also feels taken apart. When surgeons concern themselves with its particular functions, the experience is both that things are being done *to* the body and that the body is partitioned. 'Women represent themselves as fragmented – lacking a sense of autonomy in the world and carried along by forces beyond their control' (Martin 1987: 194).

Martin (1987: 201) comments on the thereby problematised function of elimination. She suggests a connection between housekeeping 'the body' of the family and women's consciousness of being grounded in a more concrete activity than men's work beyond the household gives them. Women have to manage their own bodies – including dealing with its embarrassing effluvia – as they do the household.

Let me now try to convey a different understanding of social life. To use the concreteness of certain forms to produce others implies preserving their stability; so I deploy these concepts by turning them over. Think of a culture where bodily experiences are not hidden away to be encountered as secret knowledge that resists social control, but where they are the subject of overt attention for men as well as women. And a culture which does not hypostatise 'the body' as such, for the body is not an external yet possessed presence, an integrated whole, but where on the contrary body imagery suggests social disjunction as well as conjunction. Where, indeed, every body is a composite of different identities; where bodies do not belong to persons but are composed of the relations of which a person is composed. Finally, then, a culture where partibility or fragmentation of persons/bodies is not the unintended result but as much as explicit *aim* of people's actions as is their unity.

Take the case of a people from the Central Province of Papua New Guinea who pay considerable attention to the stages of women's pregnancy and delivery.

North Mekeo comprise two endogamous tribes.[16] Within a tribe people thus think of themselves as related to one another. Yet since only 'non-relatives' can marry, the tribe is also divided into four intermarrying (exogamous) clans. Immediately after marriage, the bride

> each day is fed enormous quantities of boiled plant food along with the broth to increase the amount of womb blood in her abdomen. This sustained engorging results in a few short weeks with the bride becoming quite visibly fat. In indigenous terms, her body is also wet with plenty of skin and blood. During this time she does no work which would divert her blood away from her abdomen. Instead, she sits each day inside a mosquito net at the virtual disposal of the groom ... Through all of this, villagers say that the bride's body is 'open' (*aisekupu*). Food and drink pass from outside to inside her body in considerable quantities. As a consequence wastes, too, increase their flow from inside to outside ... Now although sexual relations are suspended upon recognition of pregnancy, the bride's body is kept 'open' with a relatively high flow of these things ... Indeed, the bride's body achieves its most 'open' condition at the moment of birth when the child emerges.
>
> (Mosko 1983: 25)

On the face of it, a culture which imposes its ideas of motherhood on the bodies of women. We are told of attendant discomforts and the woman's confinement to the house she cannot leave unchaperoned (1985: 74–5). Perversely, once conception occurs, the engorging ceases, the now pregnant woman starts eating less food and returns to work in the gardens. The forced feeding looks like a rther callow effort on men's part to metaphorise their own activity to ensure women get pregnant.

But to stop the account there would be to stop very short. It is not men who actually force-feed the bride but the groom's female relatives: they sit with her while she eats and scrutinise her development. Moreover, it is not only the bride's body which is the focus of reproductive attention. The groom's body is in synchrony. For a man's political activities are keyed into his reproductive cycle.

> His body is ... 'open' while he engages in intense procreative sexual activity with his bride. And indeed in order to sustain the steady flow ... he must eat a diet as abundant as ever he will. However, upon recognition of his wife's pregnancy the groom starts to 'close' his body ... For in the days before pacification, war was an ever-present threat. To protect ... his wife, children and other village fellows, a man had to insure that the war sorcery of enemy groups could not penetrate his body through 'open'

orifices. Also, in order to prepare his own aggressive war sorcery, a man had to 'close' his body so as not to allow the nefarious ingredients of his own charms inside. Therefore, once his wife was pregnant, the groom began ritual tightening ... This male version of closing is accomplished by sexual abstinence and the observance of complex rules of fasting with respect to food and drink. It takes some six months of this regimen to achieve a state of complete 'closing', and then the groom's body is viewed as thin, light and dry.

(1983: 26)

The diminution of the mother's diet after conception anticipates a similar process of 'tightening'. However, a woman's body remains 'open' longer than the man's:

while the mother moderates her diet, abstains from sex, and nurses the child, her body remains generally 'open'. But gradually she reverses the process; she 'closes' (*ekupu*) herself. Full 'closing' of her body is accomplished when ... she adjusts her daily regimen and weans her child at the age of one-and-a-half or two. This is the most 'closed' condition a woman can achieve. Yet it lasts only an instant, for then she is expected to reinitiate sexual relations with her husband, modifying her diet accordingly to 'open' her body again.

(1983: 25)

But if the regime still looks like the dramatic imposition of 'culture' regulating physiological rhythms, what do Mekeo make of it? What *is* the body that is the object of attention?

Let us return to the woman trying to conceive, engorging herself on food. Her surface skin becomes wet and fat. But as soon as she has a child within, this external condition changes. It is as though the woman herself is initially foetalised, her body an image of the child she is to bear. It anticipates her own transformation from being the foetus on the outside to containing the foetus within. In this sense the mother is already complete with child (= her body) before conception.[17] In fact, conception, which completes her in a different way, also starts the long process of partition by which the mother's body is de-composed, made incomplete, in the birth of the child from it.

Mekeo draw an equation between the surfaces of bodies and clans.

[There is] a metaphorical connection between the indigenous notions of 'body' (*kuma*) and clan. Indeed, villagers say of their clanswomen that they are the 'skin' (*fanga*) of the clan. Through its women or skin, the blood of a clan goes out and procreatively mixes with the bloods of other clans.

(1983: 27)

When the clan body is regarded as open to influences from others, we might say it presents a foetalised image of the women in her open state. Perhaps the foetus is thus a homology of the clan in one of its modes. For the same clan body is also open in the image of the sexually active man. The first mode indicates the clan vulnerable to influence from others, the second its ability to influence other clans. Mosko notes that just as spouses must 'close' the common boundaries of their respective bodies before beginning another child, so must clan bodies periodically unmix the bloods they have mixed and 'close' their mutual boundaries. The clan decomposes itself − extracts female members from its body − in order to make marriages with other clans; this means that the wider political unit of the tribe, composed of its constituent clans, is decomposed in turn. A woman's reproductive cycle becomes keyed into political life.

We might ask what these images exclude. (1) They forestall the idea of a linear progress from childhood to adulthood. Adult bodies cyclically return to a foetal state: the mother is made visible as the child she will carry. Yet, (2) this foetalisation is not infantilisation, a reversion to some pre-social stage. On the contrary, the image of the foetus is also the image of the widest span of political groupings, a homology of the tribe. (3) They do not present bodies as ideally in some kind of permanent state. No single form to be 'achieved', these ideas imply a constant relativisation of appearance such that one bodily form leads to another, an oscillation between composition and decomposition, between a state of completeness and making incomplete.

Completed, the body is dry, closed. Thus the newborn child moves from a wet, fat condition excreting wet faeces, to the weaned child who excretes dry ones (Mosko 1985: 81). Mother's milk, made from meat supplied by the father, 'completes' the child by externally replicating its internal constitution.

> Father and mother conceive a child with the mixing of their sexual bloods ... in equal proportions in the 'abdomen' (*ina*) of the mother. The term 'abdomen' ... is also the kin term for 'mother' (*ina*). In any case, each child receives half its hereditary blood from its father, half from its mother.
>
> (1985: 25)

The foetus/child is composed of two halves, as the entire tribe is composed of two moieties.[18] Moieties are bisected, in the same way as the child's bloods come from both its father's mother's and father's clans, and from its mother's mother's and father's clans. A microcosm of relations between four clans, it 'contains' these relations within it.

As far as 'moulding' is concerned, the child does not *look like* the tribe: it 'is' the tribe. Social relationships are not presented to the child as something to learn and acquire from the outside: for the child is there with society already within. What has to happen, in North Mekeo eyes, is that the completed child in turn must also be taken apart, for unless it becomes open it cannot enter into transactions and cannot itself conceive. As we have seen, clans internal to a tribe make themselves open to one another. This is done through prestations.

> Groom's father's clan gives valuables and pigs to bride's father's clan, and groom's mother's clan ... to bride's mother's clan ... These parallel exchanges are said to be 'manipulating blood' ... By 'manipulating blood' relatives fictiously avow that they are not relatives, that they are 'different blood' at marriage exchange ... creating the public fiction that bride and groom, with the same four clan bloods of procreation in their bodies, have instead 'different bloods' so that their marriage is legitimate.
>
> (1983: 27, transposition corrected)

Giving and receiving is an act of separation, for the two parties become distinct as donor and recipient. The result is to fragment the 'one blood' of the tribe into its components, reified in the valuables that pass out of one separately constituted body (donors) into another (recipients). As the endogamous tribe is decomposing itself, a similar transformation occurs within the bodies of its children: bride and groom.[19] Mosko introduces the metaphor of de-conception to describe that process:

> Bride and groom are ... complementarily de-conceived of their own respective grandmother's clan bloods. The groom is viewed as keeping ... only the clan bloods of his father and mother (or two grandfathers), and the bride of her father and mother (or two grandfathers) ... When the newly-weds subsequently mix their bloods in conception, their child will receive a total of only four bloods − the bloods of its four grandparents and grandparents' clans.
>
> (1983: 25)

The North Mekeo person (child/adult) thereby moves from a non-reproductive to a reproductive condition, through a process which *undoes* the act by which she or he was conceived (cf. Gillison 1987; Battaglia 1991). In order to transact with others throughout life, the body perpetually recapitulates this movement between conceived and de-conceived states.

Bodies and words

These notions do not allow, I think, the idea that things are done 'to' the body. Or rather the body is neither subject nor object, for it is as much an agent to its own compositions and decompositions as it opens to and closes itself against outside influence. Members of a tribe undo their *own* internal relations in order for marriage to take place, as a woman herself eats the food that she then releases. 'Things' are brought out from the body even as they are taken in. The body is not constructed to specifications beyond it − rather it is made to reveal what its capabilities are, is coerced to produce its own relational effects.

The succession of images allows no between: for a person or body is either the inside or outside of another person/body or else its pair form, its other half. Thus each sex presents a version of the other, like the married couple synchronising their reproductive cycles. If forms are thus conceived in an either/or mode (Munn 1986), both are always present. Nor do 'all social actors exist in situated contexts within larger spans of time−space' (Giddens 1984: 334). For space is within the actor him-/herself, as well as without. Far from empty areas being created between persons, our distances between points, gaps between the stars, North Mekeo spatiality admits extension, area, enclosure, cavity but − indeed − no voids.

Perhaps the basic issues is that Mekeo do not imagine space as infinitely receding. For what is 'beyond' the inside or outside is not more inside or outside, but an inversion or eversion of where one is at. One cannot look inside (outside) something, and then inside (outside) that, and so on through magnifications that make more inside/outside. On the contrary, what lies inside a territory is a place demarcated as an 'outside'. This is how the village looks from the point of view of the surrounding bush.[20] In Mekeo idiom, one 'goes outside' from bush (which is 'inside [the world]') to village (which is 'outside'). The outside village has at its centre its own inside place (an inverted outside). The name of this inverted outside, 'abdomen', is also used of bowels and of the womb.[21]

Outside and inside domains are bisected by such inversions because of the daily transfer of objects between village and bush (Mosko 1985: 25). The transfers include gathering food and disposal of leavings and wastes. Correlatively, faeces and urine that collect in the abdomen are already in a place outside a person's body, as we might say that the foetus inside is invertedly outside the woman's body. The womb is in this sense external to the body that encloses it, so that the sexual fluids a woman receives in its cavity remain 'outside' (1985: 89). What fills it retains that exteriority, semen and blood coming from the insides of male and female parent alike to lodge there. But like the rubbish collected in the centre of the village, or the difference between village and bush, these emissions are not moulded to the shape of the womb. They take their own different form.

This attention to bodies constitutes deliberate social practice. There is nothing inadvertent or secretive about bodily processes, including elimination, only a monitoring of when it is desirable to keep such processes within, when to reveal them. And when something is revealed, by virtue of the differentiating effect of exterior and interior, it must always take a form other than that which encloses it. Exteriority and interiority have little to do with the public/private (nor by implication political and domestic) dichotomies that concerned Martin's American women (see above). We have seen that a Mekeo body does not open to show its inner 'secret': it opens to show another, different, body.

But what is this difference? When one form displaces another, as the mother moves from being an externalised foetus to containing the foetus within her inverted outside, she alternates between two manifestations of herself. When the neonate displaces the parturient mother, its 'different form' substitutes both for her pre-pregnant body and for the pregnant body that indicates her relations with her husband. (The father becomes invisible at this point, having no contact with wife or child until weaning.) Indeed, the child is the repository of the actions of multiple others; they constitute the social relations of which it is composed. Its subsequent efforts to create 'new' ties will require altering what is already there: social activity is the dissolution and partition of completed entities. But there is nothing open-ended about this displacement. When Mekeo un-do persons (bodies) to expose the relations of which they are made, they cancel particular relations in favour of particular others. Thus a man substitutes his relations with his affines for those with his wider circle of tribal kin. But if one relation can only appear by another disappearing, it is, so to speak, prefigured or anticipated in that prior (different) form (Gillison 1991). And in that sense society is already completed.

I have, however, distorted Mosko's account. There is no indication that the person is an object of the symbolic operations he describes; even less that we can summarise Mekeo conceptions in terms of completion and lack of completion. I have translated his material this way for rhetorical effect, to contrive an analogy with Western thinking about social activity as cultural construction.

Indeed, the concept of completion is misleading if it carries resonances of a finished artefact or an ideal state. Persons alternate between states. They alternate between being a singular body of multiple composition (closed child with its four bloods) and a body bisected as one of a potential pair (open bride with 'half' her bloods; mother with internal cavity). In the latter relationships, the partner is literally completed by its pair (groom/child), completion being manifested in the relationship itself. Thus, the relations of which parents are composed are cancelled for the child to be born of *their* relationship. The one substitutes for the others, the child for its parents' procreative acts.

If in this imagery 'different' things are potentially substitutive for one another — as elsewhere, pigs are for shells, shells for brides* — then each item carries multiple references to past and future relations, and thus always to relations other than those activated in the present. Time is not infinitely receding either. Everything is present yet nothing is simply 'present'. Absence is *explicitly* anticipated/recovered, and what is absent specified, for presence is always a refiguring, a particular version. Thus only particular things can appear, and do so by showing their particular effects. From this perspective, far from everything being known (revealed), in a sense nothing is known (all is concealed), since what is apparent is only made present by its effects in specific attitudes, behaviour, bodies.

Anticipation is, so to speak, a deferral of the known. Effects emerge over time — a point many Melanesians capture for themselves through divination or omen-taking — and within persons. A woman

---

* A reference to bridewealth transactions, well documented in the ethnography of the Papua New Guinea Highlands for instance. See Chapter 6.

bears a child, but will the child be healthy? A man grows up on clan territory, but will he behave as a clansman? And people constantly scrutinise one another for evidence of their intentions, but intention is as it were the inside form of the outside actor (the presented physique, demeanour, health). While every revelation may be relativised by the previous one, each is construed as an oscillation between what is concealed and what is revealed. This means that no one form – inside or outside – holds a privileged 'constructed' place – or can reveal the deficiencies of construction. The same is true for language. The words someone speaks may be taken as one of the outward appearances he or she presents. But words too have their outsides and insides. One special province of Mekeo knowledge (of secrets and sorcery) is enclosed, even as other things can be said openly (Mosko 1985: 89). Words can be scrutinised for what they might reveal, yet this does not mean they are incomplete. The outside forms are in themselves complete: indeed they suffice as substitutes for the inside form. Thus uncertainty and doubt about others is simply the measure of oneself – not knowing what one's neighbours are up to is the external analogue of one's own internal scheming.

Literal-minded Westerners surprise themselves by finding metaphors. The discovery creates the possibility of a critique of society through language: treating texts as simultaneously literal (constructing social reality) and metaphoric (realising a social construct). Preoccupation with words themselves is part of the wider phenomenon of literalness that feminists recognise, one that prompts 'science' to know deeper and better, to see inside the bodies of things (Jordanova 1980). The problem is that we do not know how to conceal what has been revealed, reassemble what is taken apart, restore surface meanings. There 'is no whole picture that can be "filled in", since the perception and filling of a gap lead to the awareness of the gaps' (Clifford 1986: 18).

If North Mekeo seem caught up in a round of substitutions and oscillations, forever visualising themselves in alternating and anticipatory forms, then Westerners suffer a world of infinite regression. We know that the more we reveal something, the more we hide it. But our sorrow is that we always hide its inner secret. We do not see women's bodies as a form of social life; rather we see social life as hiding the body. Reveal the body and we might reveal what cannot be constructed by social life or the dominant culture! In Martin's suggestive comparison between the American woman managing the wastes of herself and the 'body' of the household, the same person does both. The household is not a version of the woman's body, but a unit of a different order. So the equation is not between a person and a set of relations, but between two different activities performed by the one person. Persons and relations, like bodies and social life, are, in the Western view, disparate phenomena.

The exhilaration of discovery for Westerners is that the further one probes, one will bring to light phenomena that will affect how one views the covering layers. Thus we un-do certain social values in order to find reasons for constructing alternative ones. Or mimic the constraints of language by pushing it to excess and thus bursting its capacity for limitation. If society distorts women's experiences, making those experiences explicit could yield a basis for a different kind of society. But this is not the only political position a Western scholar can occupy. Speaking of science, Haraway's (1988) plea for a feminist objectivity is a plea for containment of the visual gluttony of electron microscopes and satellite surveillance systems: we do not need infinite regression.

Yet regression is learned the moment we learn that culture is learned. In particular, Western investment in the metaphor of language as a carrier of culture, and of culture texted like a language, projects a counterworld of concrete individuals and natural bodies and of stubborn, non-linguistic forms. Westerners forever try to access that counterworld through composing and decomposing language itself − to trick it into revealing the unintended, to bring to speech the unspoken. The brilliance of deconstructive talk lies in its further demonstration of how such devastating counterworlds are themselves 'constructed'.

Since Melanesians compose and recompose their bodies, language simply works alongside that process with its own outsides and insides. They use language to draw attention to the analogical facility itself. Thus the manipulation of blood identities at marriage and conception are known by one Mekeo term (Mosko 1983: 29). An analogy works through the forms it juxtaposes, as bodies and words themselves are juxtaposed. Melanesians do not perform surgery on words any more than they can cut bodies open to assist birth; and do not necessarily think to expose the unintended through verbal exegesis any more than they assume that by looking inside something you will understand more about what is on the surface.

* * *

Among the images pressed into the service of critical reflection is the tenacious Western sense that experience gives individual access to a vantage point from which to apprehend the constructed nature of the world. Seen as an amalgam of conflicting and alternative elements, the internal heterogeneity of social life provides the spaces through which the critic can slip. It is not that 'individuals' and 'experiences' are free from construction themselves (clearly they are artefacts dependent on certain discourses). Rather, no *one* instance − set of values, percepts, images − is ever equivalent to the whole of perceived reality. The non-equivalence of language (or culture) to life is a starting point. By the same token, this suggests an infinite multiplication of possible forms, where refiguring must always depend on 'another perspective' (Kirby 1989: 14).

'We' thus see ourselves as caught up in complexity and diversity, through images of ever-receding knowledge and the incomplete relationship between things (society and culture) and persons (subjects, bodies). So we imagine that we shall learn more by dismantling *those forms* − undoing them to see what they are made of, an activity always proliferating, always incomplete. I have tried to make this particular form of complexity apparent through juxtaposing the practices of people who would take apart not artefacts but persons.[22] That gives them a further symbolic purchase: they use the concrete image of the body to conceal as well as reveal. They do not have to imagine a multiplying world. Things − persons − are all versions of one another: it is merely the forms that are different. Where a Westerner trying to get to the heart of something discovers a different perspective on it − yet another thing to incorporate into the schema of things − a Melanesian trying to make one thing yield something different from it produces an analogue or transformation of the original − yet another manifestation of something already present.

So if we were to look for a Melanesian counterpart to Western ideas of construction, we would have to see the generic in the particular: that any body or word is at once an entity at a particular moment in time or space (as we would say) *and*, with its past and future, its anticipation and recall of other words and bodies, is also equivalent to social life, to both genders, to all culture, to language as such. In indicating everything, such forms do not require that everything is moulded to their shape: they indicate versions of themselves that are different from themselves, as the child is 'different' from its parents' procreative acts. If so, then Melanesians such as the Mekeo

are probably not enlightened/haunted by the invisible hand of struc-
turation, that suggests we ought to, even when we cannot, decide when
acts are constraints or enablements. It would be quite exhilarating
to imagine what form, then, their politics of difference might take.

Notes

1 Geertz supposes an analogue between two anthropological practices:
anthropologists both write (thick description) and read the texts of others
over their shoulders. The second image, embedded in Geertz's (1973) own
explication of concepts of culture, caught the anthropological imagination
at the time: the first has had to be rediscovered (e.g. Bonn 1982; and the
writing stimulated by Clifford and Marcus 1986).*

2 For example, Ortner and Whitehead's (1981) subtitle is 'The cultural
construction of gender and sexuality'; Caplan's (1987) collection of essays
is called 'The cultural construction of sexuality'; see also Buckley and
Gottlieb (1988).

3 'Berger and Luckman ... demonstrated the self authenticating nature of
the social with the central ideas of reification and legitimation. Reification
referred to the way in which we forget our authorship of culture and
assign it a concrete other existence. Legitimation referred to the authority
that becomes invested in social relationships through their embeddedness
in the institutions of social structure' (Yates 1988: 14).

4 The question about whether or not cultures are perceived as complete I
derive from Roy Wagner. It is, of course, a question without which the
paper could not have been written. I also acknowledge an unpublished
manuscript of James Carrier: 'Cultural Content and Practical Meaning:
The Construction of Symbols in Formal American Culture'. The parallel
here between the child who is regarded as (in)complete and the culture
regarded as (in)complete is an example of the homology Westerners draw
between persons and society (Strathern 1988: 135, 323, etc.).

5 See Battaglia (1991).**

6 See e.g. Francesca Merlan, 'Aspects of Ritual and Gender Relations in
Aboriginal Australia', Seminar paper, Australian National University,
December 1986.

7 Wagner's (1986b) account of the provoking scepticism of the Barok of
New Ireland is pertinent here, as is Lattas's (n.d.) rendering of the Kaliai

* The metaphor of culture as a 'text' became prevalent in much anthropology in
the 1970s/80s, to be supplemented (and displaced) by a fascination with the 'cultural
construction' of texts in the mid-to-late 1980s.

** To a greater extent than the citations indicate, this essay was influenced by
Battaglia's analysis of the spaces and absences that the Melanesian Sabarl create for
themselves.

of New Britain whose verbal and ritual constructions are understood by themselves as tricks. Talk is no more nor less staged than other performances – the presentation of the 'public man' (Wagner 1987), the disclosure of acts performed (Biersack 1982), an alternative to exchange as a gesture of sociability (Strathern 1985b: 111–34). It is, therefore, not summative of them.

8 That is, undermine in this way the abstract components of which culture is 'made'.

9 For example, Fisher *et al.* (1988: 425–6): 'postmodernism is not an order constructing ideology but the deconstructive, parodic, entropic dissolution of power'; the term 'postmodern' they use ironically, *apropos* Sangren's (1988) bracketing of deconstructive and postmodernist fashions.

10 Kirby (1989: 5): 'epistemological and psychical structures of male and Western domination have provided the guarantees necessary to sustain order'; (1989: 6): 'Woman is no longer the enigma a masculinist perspective finds so fascinating ... [if] she becomes a danger to this perspective by exceeding its order'.

11 Threadgold (1988: 44, 63): 'The masculine author may be dead but the feminist *embodied* subject of liberal humanism threatens to usurp his place. Women's language will be a language which does not observe the laws of syntax. It will be characterised by a plurality of meanings and a breaking down of the unity of signifier and signified, a subversion of the notion of the unique meaning, the proper meaning of words' (1988: 62, my emphasis). Compare Harding's (1986) *deliberate* embrace of the instability of analytical categories in feminist thought.

12 'Generic norms are socially ratified situations and text-types which instantiate the sets of choices that carry dominant systems of ideas and beliefs (world-views, ideologies, epistemes) and suppress the social heteroglossia, the cultural conflict and the intertextuality out of which they are constructed. They thus reproduce and transmit the social semiotic ... *and* the contradictions and conflicts which might transform it' (Threadgold 1988: 64, original emphasis).

13. Harrison (1985); Tuzin (1982).

14. Gillison (1991); Werbner (in press).

15. Though the displacement can take place on any scale and involve a multitude of different moments of concealment and revelation.

16. My account rests heavily on Mosko's inspired 1983 paper as well as his 1985 monograph; I am also grateful for his direct comments on my rendering of his account. The Mekeo case is germane to the present argument insofar as it does *not* appear in Strathern (1988), and indeed my argument was construed independently of it. Nevertheless, I had read his book in draft form and assume that it must have written itself into my work. I take this opportunity of acknowledging its effect. The article I discovered *post hoc*.

17 The interpretation is mine. I quote Mosko's reaction (pers. com.): 'I am still unable to declare myself confidently on this one until I am certain I understand you correctly. Yes, I think it likely the prepregnant woman is being foetalized but not simply "on the outside". I would instead call particular attention to the *continuity* between the mother's wet, fat, bloody skin outside her body and [the] inverted "skin" of her womb. [The reference to an inverted interior relates to Mekeo conceptualisations of space (see below).] Both portions of skin could be seen to enclose foetuses. If so, then the mother would rather be herself invaginated by her own engorged prepregnancy skin just as her child is enclosed by the full-of-blood, folded-in skin of her womb following pregnancy but before birth. This may not be exactly what you are saying but it produces the same result nonetheless – a prepregnancy foetalized mother – and I believe in terms quite close to indigenous understandings'.

18 'The endogamous tribe, which in most contexts other than war constitutes the limit of ... Mekeo society, consists of exogamous patrilineal moieties ... each bisected into two named clans. The term for clans, *ikupu*, is in fact the nominative form of the word for 'closing' (*ekupu*) as when husband and wife "close" their bodies to one another. Each "closed" clan possesses its own estate of lands, hereditary chiefs and sorcerers, ritual paraphernalia ... [and] members of a clan or moiety distinguish themselves from, and argue their blood is "closed" to members of other clans and the opposite moiety' (Mosko 1983: 27).

19 'Bride and groom each have in their bodies the procreative (and culinary) blood of their four grandparents, and through them the blood of both moieties and all four clans of the tribe. But bride and groom derive their respective clan bloods according to distinct relationships. Blood which the groom received from father's father's clan (his own clan) his bride received from her father's mother's clan, and so on' (Mosko 1983: 27–8).

20 The perspective is non-reversible. A person going from village to bush 'goes inside'. The village is always 'outside' to the 'inside' of the bush. The relationship of inside to outside is thus relative to this spatial sequencing, as the opening and closing of social bodies is relative to the fixed number of clans.

21 Parallel to the village abdomen (an 'inverted outside'), the bush adjacent to the village is an 'everted inside'.

22 That is, they are interested in the social relations of which objects are composed, whether these objects are human beings or what human beings make or say. (In this sense they treat artefacts as persons.)

D

CHAPTER 5

Parts and wholes:
refiguring relationships

'Parts and wholes' alludes to an intellectual tradition within anthropology in which I can claim no part though it is part of the wider world in which I live.* The reason is unremarkable. Whether that world is conceptualised as British or European or Western, no one person can reproduce it in its entirety. Conversely, one cannot undo the particular processes by which one is reproduced. Or so we – whether we claim to be British or European or Western in our thinking – hold.

De Coppet (1985: 78, original emphasis) has put forward a powerful plea for the study of societies as totalities: 'Comparison is only possible if we analyse the various ways in which societies order their ultimate values. In doing so, we attempt to understand each society as a *whole*, and not as an object dismantled by our own categories'. The task is to compare not subsystems but 'societies in their own right', a holistic vision apt for 'holistic societies'. For the problem, he suggests, lies in the interference of the categories that, by contrast, reproduce 'our own individualistic society'.

If I endorse de Coppet's observation, it is to remark that conceptualisation is inevitably reconceptualisation. The society we think up for the 'Are 'Are, Melanesians from the Solomon Islands, is a transformation of the society we think up for ourselves. For instance, de Coppet says of the 'Are 'Are that far from their society's imparting its own character of permanence to the individuals who compose it, it builds up its character (of permanence) through repeated dissolution into 'the ritual and exchange process of the main elements composing each individual' (1981: 176). Instead of dismantling holistic systems

* The reference is to theorising inspired by the work of Louis Dumont, which I have never directly drawn on. I acknowledge the absence at this point by way of acknowledging the Dumontian interests of de Coppet. It was at de Coppet's invitation that I first gave the paper on which this essay is based.

through inappropriate analytical categories, then, perhaps we should strive for a holistic apprehension of the manner in which our subjects dismantle their own constructs. At least as far as Melanesia is concerned, the constructs thereby dismantled or dissolved include life-forms: persons, bodies and the reproductive process itself.

Contemporary Melanesian ethnography, especially but not only from the Austronesian-speaking seaboard, is developing its own microvocabulary of dissolution. It describes the processes by which the elements that compose persons are dismantled so that the relationships persons carry can be invested anew. This may include both the relations created during life. and the procreative (conjugal) relations that created them. A North Mekeo is 'de-conceived' first at marriage and then finally at death (Mosko 1985); Muyuw on Woodlark Island 'end' a parent's marriage when the child dies (Damon 1989); Barok mortuary feasts 'obviate' previous relationships in finally killing the dead (Wagner 1986b), a process that for the Sabarl is a 'disassembling' (Battaglia 1990) and on Gawa a 'severance' or 'dissolution' of social ties (Munn 1986). These recall Bloch's (1986) arresting account from elsewhere in the Austronesian-speaking world of the literal 'regrouping' of the dead in their tombs. But if relationships reproductive of persons sometimes have to be dissolved at death, other Melanesians see birth as the principal substitute act by which new relations displace previous ones (Gillison 1991). Indeed, all knowledge of a revelatory kind may appear as decomposition (Strathern 1988).

These counter-images to the received anthropological metaphors of structure and system have a late-twentieth-century ring to them. However, as Battaglia notes (1990: 218, n. 49), it is important to distinguish postmodernism as 'a movement with roots in the specifically historical problem of the alienating and fragmenting effects of Western socioeconomic and political influences on other cultures' from analytical perspectives (hermeneutic, deconstructivist) that have as their goal 'respect for indigenous ways of conceiving the cultural reproduction of knowledge that are themselves "perspectivist" '. Indeed, one should be as cautious as one is creative with the resonances between cultural fragmentation perceived in the world at large, specific analytical tactics such as deconstruction, and the discovery of relationships being indigenously conceptualised through images of dissolution.

The irony is that what clouds the anthropologists' holistic enterprise in the late twentieth century is no longer individualism. The 'death of the individual' has seen to that. Rather, the problem is the Western dismantling of the very category that once carried the concept of a holistic entity, that is, 'society'. Society was a vehicle for a kind of Western holism, a totalising concept through which modern people could think the holisms of others. Nowadays it seems to belong more to text than to life.[1] The modernist vision was also a pluralist one, and the pluralist vision of a world full of distinctive, total societies has dissolved into a postplural one. This is Hannerz's (1988, 1990) cosmopolitanism or creolisation, the fragmentary or hybrid global village. Yet it will no more do to shift into the vocabulary of fragmentation because of Western awareness of transnational parochialism than it was ever appropriate to export awareness of nation states or possessive individuals. At the same time, Battaglia argues (1990: 4), the new vocabulary may well capture indigenous conceptualisations that proved refractory to pluralist models.

The image of hybrid form was in fact already there in the pluralist world. It was not just the replication of like units (a multitude of distinctive but analogous societies) that pluralised anthropological vision, along with others; an equally powerful source of pluralism lay in the way different domains or orders of knowledge were brought together. Here a multitude of perspectives could pluralise the character of anything held up to study. And it is here that we find antecedents for present ideas about fragmenting parts and vanishing wholes.

This chapter is a late-twentieth-century attempt to refigure certain relationships as they have been conceptualised in this recent, pluralist past. The relationships in question belong to an apparently small domain of anthropological enquiry, those Melanesian kinship systems known as cognatic. This is because of the assumption that, despite the insignificance of kinship in Western or Euro-American society, Euro-American systems are similarly cognatic in character. Yet we cannot have it both ways; either both mode of reckoning and degree of significance are comparable or neither is. I suggest that failure to attend to the particularity of our 'own' kinship thinking has also been failure to attend to symbolic processes in anthropological thinking. It is these that have, over the last century or so, both endorsed the concept of society and dissolved it before our eyes.

The vanishing of Garia society

I start with the rebirth of a modernist paradigm. The mid-century in British Social Anthropology saw, in Kuper's phrase, a phoenix arise from the ashes. In a reconceptualised form segmentary lineage systems, as he observes (1988: 204), turned up everywhere. Among other things, they afforded a powerful equation between societies and groups.

When Lawrence finally published his account of the Garia, he rather daringly had Fortes write the foreword. It was all very well for Fortes to say that eventually the Garia concept of 'thinking on' kinsmen inspired his formulation of kinship amity. The truth is that, in 1950, Lawrence's description of these Melanesians had been a scandal. Looking back, Fortes (1984: ix) set out the problem.

> When, fresh from the field, Peter Lawrence enthusiastically described Garia social organization to me, my initial reaction was, shall we say, cautious. What later came to be designated the African segmentary descent group model was still a novelty and to many of us full of promise. Melanesia meant, above all, the Trobriands, Dobu, Manus, the Solomon Islands, and descent groups resembling those of the African Model seemed to occur in all of them. The Garia were conspicuously different ... [T]hey seemed to have a structure without boundaries: no genealogical boundaries marking off one group of people from another ... no local boundaries fixing village sites ... no political boundaries with neighbouring peoples, no closed ritual associations or exclusive access to economic resources − a society based, in short, not on unilineal descent groups but on ramifying cognatic kinship relations ... [T]his fluidity of structure posed the problem of how any sort of social continuity or cohesion could be maintained.

The only visible basis for social relations appeared to lie in the way the individual was conceived to be at the centre of radiating ties that formed a security circle.

> The essence of their social organization ... is the right of the individual to align himself ... freely with kin on the side of either of his parents ... This gives rise to the main problem that, as Radcliffe-Brown ... points out, confronts all such systems of social organization: how to counteract − how to put boundaries to − the outward extension of kinship ties to farther and farther zones of cousinship.
>
> (1984: x)

Garia social organisation was there, but where was Garia society?

Drawing on a cognatic terminology, Lawrence eventually produced a model of rights and membership. Garialand was divided into overlapping domains associated with bush gods to whom sets of persons were attached; some 200 named cognatic stocks were scattered through the domains of these gods. Each stock was presumed descended from a sibling set, internally divided between those who traced descent through males and those who traced descent through females (1984: 45). Because of certain male privileges, Lawrence also discerned patrilineages (1984: 43). He then drew on another set of Garia terms to describe an individual person's kindred. These were simply indigenous words for the closeness and distance between relatives that made a person the centre of circles of proximity. Close cognates shaded off into distant cognates, each degree of relationship including both matrikin and patrikin.

Lawrence was battling against the then prevailing cartographic images of social structure that insisted on a boundedness to the division of social interests. The concept of cognatic kinship made it appear as though it were the overlapping demands of kin alignments that created divisions. Social order was thereby apprehended as a plurality of external interests; cohesion was to be found in the security circle, where the kindred could at least be diagrammed (1984: figs 7, 9). Yet the significance of these relationships to a person was stated in a disconcertingly casual manner. 'They are merely those individuals… with whom he has safe relationships' (1971: 76).

The problems that Garia posed in 1950 were twofold. First, how to conceptualise a society that was not composed of groups; and second, the relationship of parts to wholes. If groups were the vehicles through which societies presented themselves to their members, then without group membership what was a person a part of?

The problem (for British anthropology) had been posed by Radcliffe-Brown: 'it is only a unilineal system that will permit the division of a society into separate organized kin-groups' (1950: 82).[2] Larger kin groups such as clans 'consisted of' smaller ones such as lineages (1952: 70) and lineages were composed of 'persons' such that 'the principle of the unity of the lineage group' provided a relation which linked 'a given person and all the members of the lineage group' (1952: 87). Persons could also be seen as linked in a network of kin relations that constituted 'part of that total network of social relations that I call social structure' (1952: 53). With the demonstration of structure came the assertion that between 'various features of a particular kinship systems, there is a complex relation of interdependence' such that one may conceptualise 'a complex unity, an organised whole' (1952: 53). Radcliffe-Brown could thus call for the comparison of whole systems elucidated by different kinship structures such as those manifest in lineage groups. The whole was known by its internal coherence, and thus its closure.

System, structure, group: these terms are not identical, and are not identical with society, but as a set of comprehensive, organisational categories, each provided a perspective from which that whole entity could be imagined. The recognition of groups 'by society' was further visualised in the notion that individual persons became part of society by becoming a part of a group. Descent-group theory literally focused on the mediating role of lineages and other corporate constructs in effecting social adulthood, adulthood being equated with membership. In one flight of fancy, Fortes imagined this process in the manner of a child growing from infant to adult status. The maturation of the individual is of paramount concern to society at large, he argued. Thus the domestic group 'having bred, reared and educated the child' then 'hands over the finished product to the total society' (1958: 10). As a pre-existing whole, society makes individuals into parts of itself by severing them from other pre-existing domains. Thus 'the whole society' sets itself against 'the private culture of each domestic group' (1958: 12).

If individual persons were in this mid-century view made into members of groups or of society as a whole, they were also regarded as having naturally pre-existing identities. These derived both from their biological or psychological make-up and from the domestic domain. Since domestic and politico-jural domains were conceptualised as cutting up social life into components that were not reducible to one another, each gave a different perspective on social life, and while they combined in single persons ('Every member of a society is simultaneously a person in the domestic domain and in the politico-jural domain' (Fortes 1958: 12)) they represented quite distinct relational fields. Society appeared simultaneously exclusive of and inclusive of the domestic domain. What made a person a member of society by virtue of his or her politico-jural relations was not what made him or her a member of the domestic group that supplied 'the new recruit'. In short, what gave the part ('the individual') distinctiveness as a whole person was not what made the person a part of the whole society.

The Garia problem can be rephrased: by contrast with what made a Garia a person it seemed in the 1950s impossible to discern what made a Garia a member of society.

Exchanging perspectives

Seeking the groups by which to specify membership led to much travail. But suppose the problem at which we have arrived were also a fact: suppose Garia conceived the person as a model for relationships. Instead of trying to find the groups of which a person is a member, one would then consider what modelling of relationships the person him- or herself contains. And if Garia society were modelled in the encompassing unity of the singular human being, a person would in this sense not be a part of anything else. A multitude of persons would simply magnify the image of one.

As it turned out, Lawrence placed little weight on jural relations and social cohesion. Instead he emphasised Garia pragmatism and self-interest: 'statements about moral obligation ... are no more than short-hand terms for considerations of interdependence or mutual self-interest and social survival' (1969: 29). Social conformity, he alarmingly stated, is mere by-product. A relationship valued for the practical and material advantage it confers appears subject to that person's efforts, so that even where expectation is greatest, as among close kin, any sense of indebtedness must be created. Consequently, moral obligation is limited to the circle of effective social ties. Agents thereby play an interpretive role (1984: 194) − it is they who ensure that people 'think on' them.

Lawrence's analysis of pragmatism in the conduct of relations implies no reduction to individualism. On the contrary, relations appear as significant extensions of a person's motivations: others exist in being thought upon (1984: 131ff). 'Self-regulation' thus indicates the modulation or measuring of relationships by the measure of oneself (1969: 26). He observed that it operated within the security circle, and thus tautologously with those with whom enduring and effective ties could be demonstrated. Iteanu (1990) offers a similar observation for Orokaiva. People make relationships specific to themselves. External relations are centred on persons as at once subjects and objects of the multiple configuration of their acts, inclinations and judgements.[3]

In Western terms it would seem a paradox that relationships are not mapped as external connections among a plurality of individuals. Instead, the singularity of the Garia person is conceptualised as a (dividual) figure that encompasses plurality. If in the Garia view there are no relationships that are not submitted to the person's definition of them, then what the person contains is an apprehension of those relations that he or she activates without. If they pre-exist, it is as internal differences within his or her composite body. This I believe is also an image of the 'group'. Garia conceptualisations suggest that whatever sociality constitutes the person also constitutes the manner in which relations compose the stock or bush god territories. They are all homologous (Mosko 1985) persons ('beings', de Coppet 1985). In this sense, what makes up the part also makes up the whole. As a result, a collectivity such as a cognatic stock is neither an aggregate nor sociality of a different order and can appear equally as one person or as many persons. In the manner, then, in which Garia persons are conceptualised as managing their relations with others, they are the equivalent of all the relationships focused on them.

So what do we do with the recurrent internal division of persons into male and female elements? In their figure of the kindred, focused on a living sibling set with its constellation of maternal and paternal kin, or the bush god territory, focused on an ancestral sibling set with access divided between male- and female-born, Garia conceptualise a composite, androgynous person. I wish to suggest that what distinguishes Garia formulations from the familiar groupings of the so-called lineal systems of their neighbours lies in a temporal modality. What is at issue is the divisive figuring of gender to create a future image of unity.

The point at which persons appear as a composite of male and female elements and the point at which a single gender is definitive are also temporal moments in the reproduction of relations that take a mode imagined across all of Melanesia.[4] Unity emerges once a dual gender identity has been discarded in favour of a single one. The process entails an oscillation between the person conceived as androgynous and the person conceived as single-sex – as when groups from elsewhere in Papua New Guinea conceptually shed members of one sex (in marriage) in order to reconceive themselves as 'one person' composed of the members of the other. Single-sex persons are presented through the bodies of men or of women or through the mobile female or male items of wealth that pass between them.

The decomposition of the composite person thereby reveals the relations, at once internal and external, of which he or she is composed.

Such a Melanesian person – androgynous or single-sex – is not some kind of corporation sole, and the singular person is not conceptualised as a group with relations extrinsic to it. The matrilineal Trobriands, whom Fortes so eloquently claimed for descent-group theory, present a case in point.

Throughout their lifetimes, Trobrianders activate relationships in a mode that makes the form that every living person takes a composite by maternal and paternal kin. The person can be conceptualised as a vessel, like a canoe containing matrikin, adorned on the outside of its relations with others and especially relations through men. Indeed, the entire kula exchange system is a kind of adornment to matrilineality. At death, the person is divided and, as Annette Weiner (1976, 1979, 1983) has shown, the descent group achieves unitary form as a collection of ancestral spirits waiting to be reborn. This is a moment at which it appears as a single-sex entity – as it also appears in the images of land or of blood that contain the living body. When it takes after the living person, however, the descent group appears in the form of its numerous extensions and relations to others: land attracts sons to stay and the foetus is nourished by the father.

Whether external or internal, relations are intrinsic not extrinsic to the living person (Wagner 1991). One might say that relations are what animates the person – vividly imagined in the Trobriand canoe that speeds across the water because of its masculine attributes, towards partners created through paternal and affinal ties. If relationships give a person life, then at death what is extinguished are those relationships embodied by the deceased. Indeed, a significant effect of Massim mortuary ceremonies is to strip the deceased of social ties: the enduring entity is depersonalised. Relationships created during the lifetime are thus refashioned, for the living can no longer embody them. In some cases (e.g. Mosko 1989; Battaglia 1990), it is as though people had to recompose the world as it was before the person existed. But it can only be recomposed in other persons. The cognatic entity built up during a lifetime is partitioned at death.

The neighbouring Molima of Fergusson Island (Chowning 1989) also separate paternal and maternal kin after death. Like the Garia, the Molima kinship system would have to be called cognatic. Yet the relative lack of differentiation among consanguines holds only during an individual's lifetime. At death, the body of kin dissolve into those whose ties to the deceased are through women and those whose ties are through men.[5] The kin of the deceased divide themselves into mourners and workers, each category becoming conceptually single-sex (as children of a brother, children of a sister). Yet such a division is a general not a special state of affairs in Melanesia. It is not that cognatic systems are aberrant[6] but that everywhere in this part of the world the composite person is a cognatic system, to be undone or otherwise depluralised, transformed into a unitary entity at particular moments in time. It is simply that Molima do not realise their antici-pations of this moment until they assemble to do mortuary service.

In short, what anthropologists have classified as differing principles of Melanesian social organisation can also be understood as an effect of modalities in temporal as well as spatial sequencing. The mode of dissolution is various, but the 'social organisation', the person, is similarly construed everywhere. To apprehend this, we need to ap-prehend the nature of Melanesians' 'perspectivism'. For they live in a world in which perspectives take a particular form, namely, that of analogies. The result is that perspectives can be exchanged for one another.

During a lifetime, a singular person exists as an integral part of relations, if we wish to figure it that way; but only in the sense that the part is made from the same material as the whole. Relations also appear as an integral part of persons – the Garia security circle being managed by people's dispositions, the Trobriand descent group with its outward extensions towards others. What makes the person, then, is no different from what makes up these relations.

Nonetheless, relations appear at different times and in different locations. This is where perspective becomes important. A male member of a matrilineage is both like and unlike a female member, a collectivity of men giving birth to an initiate is both like and unlike a solitary woman in labour, the yams that swell the belly of the Trobriand brother's garden are both like and unlike the yams with which a father feeds his children. There is constant diversification of the forms in which persons and relations appear. Indeed, one may turn into another: my sister is your wife. These are switches of per-spective between the positions that persons occupy: donor becomes recipient, daughter's paternal substance becomes mother's maternal substance. A temporal perspective is evident, for instance, in the patrilineal clan groups of the Papua New Guinea Highlands. The groups exist in anticipation of action, the spatial reminders of clan unity – men's house, territorial boundary – expectant of the moment when the clan will act as one. As one body, one gender, the clan in turn will act to dispose or rearrange the focus of others in relation to it. A clan is thus a transformation of other relations in a specific spacetime (Munn 1986). The 'cognatic' or androgynous person becomes depluralised, decomposed, in the creation of the 'unilineal' single-sex person. Heterogeneous internal relations are thus everted, and appear to the agentive clan(sman) as the network of external affines and consanguines it can focus on itself.

In these cases, an oscillation of temporal perspective (before/after) may be imagined as a substitution of external for internal form, or of the gender of persons. In the case of gender, a double perspectival move is possible between male and female and between same-sex and cross-sex relations. Yet if these are perspectives they have interesting properties. Instead of providing the bases from which to conceive radically different worlds of knowledge, Melanesian forms allow perspectives to exist at once as analogues and as (potential) transformations of one another. For they contain the possibility that persons can exchange perspectives. My centre is not your centre, but your detached sister/brother (wealth) can be incorporated as the mother/father of my children (my means of reproduction). What is not at issue is that switch of perspective required to perceive an individual as an entity differently constituted from the relationships of which it is part. It is impossible, for instance, to imagine a person cut out from relations and remaining alive (cf. Leenhardt 1979 [1947]). A person is only divested of relations when it no longer embodies them.

In the way that Melanesians present social life to themselves, it would seem that there are no principles of organisation that are not also found in the constitution of the person. External relations have the same effect as internal ones. In short, to imagine the person in this manner means that no switch of perspective between person and relations is required in order to 'see' social relations. Exchanging perspectives only differentiates one set of relations from another, as it does one kind of person from another.

Cognatic kinship?

No more than 'society', however, will this figuring of the person do as a simple cross-cultural category. It is inadequate in turn for grasping the worlds that Euro-Americans imagine for themselves. However, it is an instructive figure with which to conceptualise the difference.

It may seem curious to resurrect British descent-group theory of the mid-century when other – largely Continental – formulations of the time were based on the premise that persons have relations integral to them (what else is the specification of the positive marriage rule?), but I do so to remark that at its core was an interesting symbolic device. The nature of the debate that it precipitated over non-unilineal kinship systems reveals in retrospect the character of an indigenous Euro-American kinship system – less in the classification of relations it purported to offer than in the conceptualisation of kinship with respect to society. The English are my example, and I take an insider's view.[7]

The matter can be put simply. The English person conceptualised as an individual was in one important sense incomplete (after Carrier n.d.). There always appeared to be 'more than' the person in social life. When the singular person was taken as a unit, relationships involved others as like units. Social life was thus conceptualised as the person's participation in a plurality. As a result, an individual person was only ever a part of some more encompassing aggregate, and thereby less than the whole. Where a prototypical Melanesian might have conceptualised the dissolution of the cognatic person as making incomplete an entity already completed by the actions of others, our prototypical English took the person – powerfully symbolised in the child that must be socialised – as requiring completion by society. To focus on the individual person inevitably dissolved this larger category, fragmenting the 'level' at which holism could be seen. Radcliffe-Brown called for the comparison of whole systems because (from the point of view of systems) only systems were whole. The English paradox was that holism was a feature of a part – not the whole – of social life! That is, it was a feature more evident from some (e.g. systemic) perspectives than from others. A particular property of such perspectives was that they appeared either as irreducibly plural or as 'more' or 'less' totalising or partial.

That the English imagined themselves living between different orders or levels of phenomena, in an incommensurate world of parts and wholes, both created and was itself a precipitate of the manner in which they handled perspective. I have suggested that an example of this way of thinking was evident in the mid-century British debates over cognatic kinship.

Unilineal descent groups were taken as evincing the characteristics of orderly social life. Above all, membership could be demonstrated. Indeed, in their kinship organisation, many non-Western peoples seemed to be doing what the anthropologist was also doing in elucidating social structure: classifying according to conventions of social life. The individual person was situated within an order of sociality – descent and succession – whose identity clearly endured beyond the life of any one member. 'Life' as such became an attribute of abstract social systems (Fortes 1958: 1). From the perspective of descent, a group could be conceptualised as a (single) juristic person (Fortes 1969: 304). Yet, as we have seen, the same argument assumed that what made individual persons members of a whole group was not what made them whole persons.

Social life was understood as convention. If convention or classification demarcated sociality, then a particular significance seemed to inhere in those parts of the kinship system that regulated the disposition of assets, the loyalty of members, and their own definition as sociocentric entities. Hence the significance of the distinction between 'descent' and 'kinship' and between those (politico-jural) relations that affected group affiliation and those focused on ego as an individual. To the extent that the first set of relations appeared social, the second appeared based on natural connections. The domestic domain was thus seen to deal with reproduction as a biological necessity; there was an internal logic to its own developmental cycle (Mosko 1989), and the network of kin ties focusing on the individual ego appeared a natural ground to other kin conventions. 'Society' and 'nature', we might say, mapped different domains of social relations, the former being more obviously moulded by convention than the latter.[8]

Indeed, consanguineal relations as such indicated a virtual fact of nature, a universalism in human arrangements. There were, it seemed, no societies that, in taking account of parentage, did not take account of the presence of both maternal and paternal kin: 'filiation ... is universally bilateral' (Fortes 1970 [1953]: 87). Recognition of consanguinity was unremarkable. What varied was the extent to which kin relations were the social basis for group membership. British Social Anthropology became preoccupied not only with types of descent, but with whether peoples had descent groups at all.

It is a pity that the term 'cognatic' should have been so emphatically developed as a complement to the lineal 'agnatic' or 'uterine'.[9] Cognatic ties, wrote Fortes (1970 [1943–4]: 49) are 'ties of actual or assumed physical consanguinity'. For Tallensi, it is in the domestic family that we have 'the sharpest picture of the interaction between cognatic kinship and agnatic ties. We have there the elementary ties of cognatic kinship linking parent to child and sibling to sibling, and we also have the agnatic tie which sets apart the males as the nuclear lineage' (1970 [1943–4]: 50). Cognatic kinship thus emerged as a kind of ground against which the social relations based on agnation appear. The creation of the latter came to look like the creation of society (out of nature).[10] One may depict it thus: (1) Descent groups exemplified the creation of *social difference* – bounded sociocentric entities cut out of the ramifying networks of individuals. Society was evident in conventional differentiation. (2) The field of cognatic kin thus appeared as a set of consanguines *naturally undifferentiated* – the raw material of kinship. In descent-group systems non-lineal cognates were acknowledged through complementary filiation or the residual claims of subsidiary ties.

The term 'cognatic' was unfortunate if only in that it was in use, and had been for a century (Freeman 1961), for those many other systems in which unilineal descent groups did not exist at all. The prototypes were European as well as English.[11] Without unilineal privilege, each parent was of equal weight and equally differentiated. What became interesting was the effort anthropologists put into redeeming the social significance of kin ties in such societies. The question was how you could both have cognatic systems and have groups. It seemed commonly the case that cognatic kin-reckoning coexisted with cutting or bounding classifications that rested on other-than-kinship criteria such as residence (cf. Scheffler 1985). Cognatic systems thus came to have a dual theoretical status, marginalised both in relation to lineal systems and in terms of their own internal kinship constructs. The latter seemed either thoroughly uninteresting or else thoroughly familiar. Interest lay rather in the (non-kinship) conventions by which such systems achieved the kind of closure necessary if they were to be, in the parlance of the time, the building blocks of society.

This focus had been built into kinship studies by the American Morgan. His 'descriptive' systems were a kind of terminological counterpart to cognatic kin-reckoning, and ones that purported to describe the world as it was. Such kin terminologies 'correctly' discriminated among given discriminations in the world: in Kuper's (1988: 56) critical comment, they 'mirror[ed] the reality of biological kinship'. After all, terms describing natural differences preserved the uniqueness and particularity of parentage. It was the conventions of other systems that cut the natural facts artificially, classifying relatives in a way that anthropological expertise must then untangle. The 'classificatory' or 'artificial' system certainly did not tell the world as it was. Rather, it 'confound[ed] relationships which, in their nature, are independent and distinct' (quoted in Trautmann 1987: 138).

As a result, descriptive systems appeared to display neither artificiality nor convention. If the descriptive system did not need explanation by reference to social convention, its terminologies could be mapped directly onto (natural) relations of consanguinity. To later anthropologists it seemed therefore that one hardly needed social theory to understand it. This was a drastic assumption, for by the mid twentieth century convention had become the object of study, and the problems for untangling appeared all the other way. Kinship systems that produced groups were no trouble. The trouble with cognatic systems was that tracing cognatic kinship could neither in a strong sense produce groups nor in a weak sense yield a sense of convention or society. Here, in the absence of lineality, was the inverse case: (1) Cognatic kinship reflected *natural difference* in the bilateral reckoning of relations. (2) But the field of cognatic kin was thus *socially undifferentiated* and groups had to be cut out of this field by criteria of a different order.

Society, like the analyses anthropologists produced, was to be made visible in its internal differentiations and categorisations, the social segments it cut from nature. Yet in the cognatic case one saw only the endless recombination of elements devolved from and focusing on individuals. Natural proliferation, ties stretching for ever: as Fortes voiced in his comments on the Garia, there seemed no structure to the mode of kin-reckoning itself. Even when kin categories could be identified as focused on sibling pairs or married couples, the result was overlapping and thus incomplete classifications. Conceptualised as a kind of inverse to lineal holism, the workings of cognatic kinship seemed incapable of yielding a model of a whole.

If 'society' were most visible in groups, it was because they too exemplified classification and convention. For society was held to inhere in the 'level' of organising principles, not in what was being ordered; levels were literally conceived as of a different order from persons concretely imagined as so many individuals. Hence the central problematic of mid-century anthropology: the relationship between individual and society. Each comprised an irreducible perspective on the other, and the result was pluralism. To think of society rather than to think of the individual was not to exchange perspectives, for there was no reciprocity here. Rather, it was to switch between totalising worlds. Here each perspective encompassed the other perspective as 'part' of itself.

In this presentation of part–whole relations, the whole was composed of parts, yet the logic of the totality was to be found not in the logic of the individual parts but in organising principles and relations lying beyond them. To perceive life from the perspective of the discrete parts thus yielded a different dimension from the viewpoint gained from the whole. Depending on what was taken as a whole and what was taken as a part, one could always generate (whole) new perspectives and new sets of elements or components. Each part was potentially a whole, but only from other perspectives. Thus an individual person was a potentially holistic entity – but, for anthropologists, only from the perspective of another discipline such as psychology. From anthropology's own disciplinary perspective, the concept of society stimulated the 'more' holistic vision.

The vanishing of English kinship

To argue that the symbolic strategy at the heart of this kinship theorising was based on the idea that parts cannot be defined by what defines wholes, recalls Schneider's (1968) formulation of American kinship. What makes a person a relative, he stated, is not what makes a relative a person. It is to such a switch of perspectives that the kinship constructs of the mid twentieth century gave facticity and certainty. What was embedded in anthropological kinship thinking was, I suspect, reflected back by the folk models of the 'wider society' of which it was a part.

Now while I take 'English' as my exemplar of a folk model and thus illustrative of Euro-American kinship thinking, there is also good reason to suppose that the trivialisation of kinship in social life is a characteristic that may well distinguish it from some continental or southern European models (though it may give it an affinity to aspects of 'American' kinship). It is of interest insofar as it has helped shape British anthropological theorising on kinship. Both belong to a cultural era I have called 'modernist' or 'pluralist'.

The short question is why a kinship system of the English kind has been so hard to conceptualise theoretically. Part of the answer must lie in conceptualising it as cognatic. For that meant it became profoundly uninteresting. Either its mode of kinship reckoning is entirely unproblematic because it self-evidently follows natural distinctions or it is entirely problematic because it solves so few of the other questions we would ask about social life. It disappears in studies of local communities or class or visiting patterns. We have a feeling that kinship in English society ought to have a significant social dimension, despite the fact that all we can see is the number of times daughters visit their mothers or who gets what at Christmas. But what we then 'see' is the incompleteness of kinship as an explanatory device. We reintroduce dimensions of class and income and neighbourhood and our grasp of what might be distinctive about kinship has again vanished.

That the English cannot pin down a sense of society when they reflect on their own kinship systems is an artefact of the system itself. And that is because of the way they make kinship vanish. Collaterals do not, of course, go on forever; they fade out rather quickly (Firth *et al.* 1969: 170–1), but not for reasons to do with the nature of the kin connection. Other factors intervene; and this is the point. Kinship seems less than a complete system. 'Kinship and marriage', Fox (1967: 27) writes, 'are about the basic facts of life. They are about "birth, and copulation, and death".' But birth and copulation and death are not about society. Rather, they chart the individual person's movement 'through' it. Fox expresses this common-sense disjunction in an unremarked shift of phrase. 'Birth produces children ... Death produces a gap in the social group.'

From a British view, then, despite our best efforts as anthropologists to see our own conventions, we somehow take the manner in which the English (say) trace kin along lines of consanguinity as socially trivial. Society lies 'beyond' kinship, impinging as a different order of phenomena. But suppose that this problem were also fact: suppose that this incompleteness were part of English kinship thinking. Instead of trying to specify what the social significance of kinship might be, we would consider what modelling of plurality kinship formulations themselves contain. Let me rephrase the modelling at issue and reinstate the tense that indicates the temporal perspective from which I write.

What I have called modernist or pluralist in this kinship thinking produced the figure of the person as an individual, made up of the physical materials that made up other individuals but recombining them in a unique way. In this sense, the person was a whole individual. But what made the person a whole individual was not what made him or her a part of any wider identity. In relation to society, the individual was incomplete – to be completed *by* socialisation, relationships and convention. The problematic at the heart of mid-century British anthropology was also a proposition at the heart of twentieth-century English kinship.

The proposition neatly encapsulated the manner in which anthropologists produced plural and fragmented worlds for themselves as much as it did the manner in which they produced totalising and holistic ones. For the moment one switched from looking at a person as a unique individual to his or her relations with others, one added a dimension of another order. Each perspective might be used to totalising effect, yet each totalising perspective was vulnerable to other perspectives that made its own purchase on reality incomplete. The individual person was both a part of society and a part of nature. Society both was cut out of nature and encapsulated nature within itself. To switch from one perspective to another was to switch whole domains of explanation. The parts were not equal since perspectives could not be matched. They overlapped; one whole was only a part of another. Thus social convention could be conceptualised as modifying and encompasing natural givens; and what made up the elements of a narrative was not conceptualised as the narrative itself.

This was evinced in the biology of procreation and death. A child was endowed with material from both parents, literally formed from parts of them. Yet it was regarded as equivalent to neither mother nor father, nor to the relation between them: rather, it was a hybrid product in another sense, a genetically unique individual with a life of its own. It was only a part of their life, despite the fact that its genetic material was formed wholly from theirs. On the other hand, at death, what gave the individual uniqueness was left as the acts and relations exercised during the lifetime – the individual person only borrowed a part of life itself. Like society, life would carry on. So now life was part of the individual person, now the individual was a part of life: life and person overlapped but did not match. Built into this conceptualisation was a generative incompleteness. If genetic endowment must be complemented by environment and nurture, there was no sense in which a kinsperson could stand for a social totality.

A consequence of such thinking was that once a foetus was created through the recombination of genetic elements, that conception could not be undone. Similarly, a person always retained social identity, as an individual with a life history, and this remained true after death. Death did not take away the individuality of the person. What it did, though, was take away life.

Life was regarded, then, as larger than the person who embodied it. The deceased was colloquially 'cut off' from a stream of existence that was more than him or her, as he or she was cut off from an active part in social relationships. Death terminated the enjoyment of relations, such as marriage, that remained thereafter frozen in the record (cf. Wolfram 1987: 213). People also spoke of persons in their lifetime 'cut off' from society, or even 'cut off' from their kin – by which they meant not the undoing of genetic inheritance but separation from a domain of sociability. Indeed, 'rootlessness' applied to persons signified less a change in the nature of physical attachment to others than the state of being cut off from a community of persons, typically from home. Kin could thus be seen as a kind of community, a background from which the striving individual might seek to depart.

The kinsperson, in this mid-century view, recombined genetic material in irreversible sequence. But when he or she was thought of as cut out of something, that something appeared as a metaphysical entity of a different order of reality from the person: society, home, even life itself. In fact, death most concretely indicated that whatever it was that the individual person belonged to in his or her lifetime, it was only the individual deceased who ceased to be part of it; that other something continued.

Such modernist perspectives had their own pluralising effect. When perspectives cannot be exchanged, one perspective can only capture the essence of another by encapsulating it as a part of itself. Parts in turn thus always appear to be cut from other, larger wholes. But if perspectives cannot be imagined at all, what then?

Postplural visions

Some people in the West think they now live in a world that has lost the unifying perspective of modernism. This leaves the problem of what to do with parts and wholes. I offer an American example.

I have been struck by the organising images of Clifford's *The Predicament of Culture* (1988), his concern with the rootlessness that offcentres persons and scatters traditions. This mood of lost authenticity − the idea that the world is full of changed, part-cultures − is not new. What is new (he says) is the setting that the late twentieth century provides: 'a truly global space of cultural connections and dissolutions has become imaginable: local authenticities meet and merge in transient ... settings' (1988: 4). The task is how to respond to an unprecedented overlay of traditions. Ethnography must be an ethnography of conjunctures, moving between cultures, a cosmopolitan practice which participates in the hybridisation he sees everywhere. Yet (he argues) ethnographies have always been composed of cut-outs, bits extracted from context, brought together in analysis and narrative. What is also new is the way we think about the hybridisation. Texts that once celebrated the integration of cultural artefacts have been displaced by deliberate attention to the uniqueness of fragments. Creativity can only lie in their recombination. Clifford sees this as a salvation not just for texts but for the concept of culture itself, for cultures have always been hybrids, 'the roots of tradition [forever] cut and retied' (1988: 15). Tradition?

The therapeutic hope of his own efforts is for the 'reinvention of difference' (1988: 15). Elements cut from diverse times and places can be recombined, though they cannot fit together as a whole. He back-projects the supposition that they never did. So he is left with another problem, which is what on earth they have been cut *from*. Distinctive ways of being still exist despite their hybrid manifestations and he evokes the shadowy presence of some other dimension, rather like a lost perspective. Now, Clifford is coy about characterising this dimension − this realm of an order different from the individual fragments yet from which the fragments have come. No doubt he is coy for the reason that his predecessors have been certain, for he does not want to reconceptualise a totalising whole.

Clifford's problem, then, is not that of simple multiplicity or of the multiculturalism of contact. Rather, it is a postplural vision of a composite world forever the result of borrowings and interchanges.

In his view, such a habitation significantly resists the global vision of (say) Lévi-Strauss's *Tristes tropiques* (1955), with its 1950s nostalgia for authentic human differences disappearing in an expansive commodity culture. Rather than being placed at the end of the world's many histories, the European narrative of a progressive monoculture is to be set beside the creolisation of culture itself. He evokes the Caribbean: a history of degradation, mimicry, violence, but one that is also rebellious, syncretic and creative. Without wholes, the only thing to do is recombine the parts.

Listen, then, to how the images of recombination and cutting work. Listen to what happens when one imagines Clifford's vision of the postmodern world as though he were thinking kinship of the English kind.

Clifford's criticism is of those who mistook people's collections for the representation of a collective life: there never were any authentic indigenous master narratives for which the anthropologist's master narrative was an appropriate genre. The classifier of ethnographic collections 'invents' a relationship between artefact and culture. Cut out of their (living) contexts, artefacts are made to stand for abstract wholes, a Bambara mask for Bambara culture. Creolisation, by contrast, makes incongruity evident, as in ethnographies which leave 'the cuts and sutures of the research process' visible (1988: 146). Ethnography as collage 'would be an assemblage containing voices other than the ethnographer's, as well as examples of "found" evidence, data not fully integrated within the work's governing interpretation' (1988: 147). Here is the potential creativity of ethnography. Rather than the creativity of convention, of human kinship 'reduced to discrete differential systems' (1988: 241), ethnography must remain open to registering the original act of combination – the procreation of a hybrid.

Clifford's presentation of cultures as bits and pieces cut up and recombined contains borrowings of its own. Let me recapitulate. On the one hand, like rootless persons cultures are always in fragments; on the other hand in their collecting it is part anthropologists who have cut up cultures into the bits reassembled in their narratives. Cultures are always hybrids, yet cultural future lies in further creative recombining, including the recombinations of the ethnographic enterprise. As Clifford depicts the late-twentieth-century ethnography, its skilled differentiations will apply to differences already there. He quotes Said: 'A part of something is for the foreseeable future going to be better than all of it. Fragments over wholes ... To tell your story in pieces, *as it is*' (1988: 11, original emphasis).

This is the old reproductive idiom of biological kinship. Clifford does not, of course, talk kinship. Yet transmuted into his language of ethnographic creativity are, I suggest, ideas equally applicable to mid-century notions of procreation. Persons are natural hybrids: the creative recombination of already differentiated genetic material makes everyone a new entity. The past might have been collected into ancestral traditions, but the future lies in perpetual hybridisation.

That genetic analogy was not available to Morgan, but the manner in which Morgan's descriptive systems distinguish own parents from collateral relatives emphasises the particulate state of each individual. The particularity of parentage is the guarantee (cf. Schneider 1984). Thus genealogical trees appropriately focus on ego, the individual repository of inheritances recombined from other persons, each in turn unique. It was this particularism that classificatory terminological systems with their artificial conventions failed to describe. If there were a sense in which descriptive terminologies seemed self-evident to Morgan, I see a devolved parallel with Clifford's late-twentieth-century vision. Clifford finds it unproblematic to convey the hybridisation of a hybrid world, with its particulate nature and unique moments. Yet hybrids are not to be stabilised as wholes. For him, all the 'problems' lie in those master narratives which purported to reveal holistic societies – in which case the real problem lies in being heir to them, and thus to the supposition that parts are always cut from something else: how to conceptualise a part that is not a part of a whole?

From Morgan to Clifford might seem a bizarre genealogy, but these figures are useful bookends. Morgan belonged to an era that had just finished debating whether humankind had one or many origins; Clifford speaks for a world that has ceased to see either unity or plurality in an unambiguous way. What lie between are those years of modernist scholarship with their vision of a plurality of cultures and societies whose comparison rested on the unifying effect of this or that governing perspective. Each perspective simultaneously pluralised the subject matter of anthropological study and held out the promise of a holistic understanding that would show elements fitted together and parts completed.

At least for British anthropology, I suspect it was a similar intimacy between anthropological and folk models that in fact made the indigenous system impossible to analyse; it either appeared as a negative version of other kinship systems, or was universalised as displaying the facts that others tried to conventionalise. Such conventions were found in societies where kinship seemed central to the manner in which society itself was represented. 'Kinship' was, of course, already conceptualised as a 'system', and systems were seen to be wholes made up of (interdependent) parts. But to give 'parts' their distinct identity would draw one into other perspectives, other totalising systems of relations. In Western society one could take the perspective of kinship but this could not also be the perspective of society.

In anthropological discourse, systems, like conventions or like societies and cultures, were frequently personified as agents with interests of their own – an image laminated in the depiction of corporate groups as juristic persons. But perhaps Clifford does more than reconceptualise an old procreative model. His postplural vision repersonifies relationships as a living hybrid of forms, so that all that is visible is culture itself – the grafting process of cultivating new growth from previous material. Perhaps his vocabulary also looks forward to a new kinship that will have to deal with transgenic life-forms and the mapping of the human genome in the interest of therapy. If so, it is a vocabulary suffused with nostalgia for an unproblematic holism.

Think again of the Garia person. It was a fancy, of course, ever to have supposed that this Melanesian figure contains an image of 'society', for the very idea of society in Western thinking entailed an encompassment of perspectives. Society did not in Garia modelling provide a perspective on the singular person any more than the singular person provided a perspective on society. There was in that sense no perspective; or, rather, only the one perspective, from the centre, of which others were always analogies or transformations. Thus to imagine another person was to exchange perspectives: one person's periphery appeared as another person's centre (Werbner, in press). But is one perspective not also a loss of perspectives? Whatever insight a postplural vision might yield here, Garia nostalgia is unlikely to be of the English or American kind.

New dismantling idioms might give anthropologists a vocabulary with which to apprehend other people's dismantling projects but 'our' project should not be mistaken for 'theirs'. We are not devolved from and do not reproduce the same worlds.

Parallels between 'Melanesian' and 'Western' conceptualisations always were elusive. The Garia security circle looked at first blush like the ramifying kin network of consanguines with which many Europeans were familiar. Yet the figure of the Garia person was never a genetic hybrid, complete by inheritance and endowment but incomplete when thought of as a part of a wider society. Rather, socially complete, it was made incomplete in its engagement and exchange with others. Nor did the holism of Melanesian imagery mean that Melanesians did not envision cutting. On the contrary, images of partition, extraction, severance were commonplace. Differentiation was a principal preoccupation (see e.g. J. Weiner 1988): male from female, donor from recipient, the protocols were endless. But what was 'cut' were persons and relations themselves: person from person, relation from relation, not persons cut off from relations. Far from being fixed in time at the moment of birth, relations were the active life on which the person was forever working.

What differentiated relations in Melanesia was the exchange of people's perspectives on one another: the transfer of valuables that guaranteed that a woman would bear her husband's child and not her father's or the work of spouses in procreation that must be repeated before birth and supplemented by nurture afterwards. A person was created, so to speak, out of the same materials by which it created its own life: composite but not unique; 'cut' and partitioned but not from a sphere that lay external to it. The Highlands woman being prepared for marriage might be both severed from her clan and internally divided – detached from and made to void paternal substance. Everything was partible.[12] But this partitioning did not create different orders of being out of parts and wholes.

The modernist imagery of parts and wholes worked to different effect, and it is to this that we are heir. It made us see persons as parts cut from a whole imagined as relations, life and, for the anthopologist, society. Conversely, in the discourse of systems and structures it was relations, life, society that creatively recombined the fragments and parts. The 'cognatic kinship' of Western society reproduced unique individuals whose procreation was perpetually modified by an overlay of other principles of social life. Take the individual away and, English would say, society will still endure. But a Melanesian death required the active severance of persons and relations – living persons rearranging their relationships among themselves when the deceased could no longer embody them. This included 'undoing' the cognatic ties which constituted life.

What was creative about the recombinations that Melanesians enacted – the wealth and children they made – was that they anticipated and were made of acts similar to those which subsequently partitioned them. Parts were never dislocated in this sense, left on the cutting-room floor, so to speak, to be recombined by someone else. Contrary to understood wisdom, Melanesians have never needed salvage ethnography. For their vision of the world had no problem with how parts fit together. There were no bits and pieces that had to be put back again, for the sake of a culture to restore, a society to conceptualise. Saved Clifford's predicament, I doubt that nostalgia for either culture or society figures in their present cosmopolitanism.

Notes

1 For instance, Thornton argues that much of the significance of 'society' lay in its power as a rhetorical trope for the organisation of anthropological data. Positing analytical components capable of theoretical integration presumed an entirety to the object of study as a whole made up of parts, so that society emerged as a holistic precipitate of analysis. 'The imagination of wholes is a rhetorical imperative for ethnography since it is this image of wholeness that gives the ethnography a sense of fulfilling "closure" that other genres accomplish by different rhetorical means' (1988: 286). Conversely, 'it may be that it is impossible to conceptualize society, except in terms of holistic images' (1988: 298). Analysis in turn became the decomposition of an imagined whole. Outside the Dumontian tradition, much of the convincing character of society as a whole derived from the equally convincing representation of parts ('subsystems') that could be further subdivided into parts.

2 While Fortes (1970 [1953]: 81) allowed himself to refer to '[a] society made up of corporate lineages', it was an image that he later took great pains to undo (e.g. 1969: 287). On the disjunction between Fortes's own rich documentation of the Tallensi case (including their overlapping fields of clanship) and his theoretical axioms, see Kuper (1982: 85); and for a similar point with regard to the relationship of 'descent' and 'group', see Scheffler (1985: 9).

3 I do not make here a distinction offered elsewhere (Strathern 1988: Ch. 10), between persons as the objects of relations and agents who act in respect of persons/relations.

4 What renders the so-called lineal systems distinct is the way in which relations engaged in the lifetime are regarded as making the complete

lineage person 'incomplete' -- the person is restored to a final completeness (a state of pre-procreation) at death.

5 On Molima, the mortuary rearrangements of persons are permanent but cannot take place in advance; elsewhere they are anticipated and may even be acted upon in pre-mortuary exchanges finalised at death. In the Papua New Guinea Highlands, birth is the prominent event in relation to which people dispose themselves, entailing the fresh affirmation of relations on a categorical basis, above all the distinction between the child's paternal and maternal kin.

6 'Cognatic systems' crop up all over Melanesia with disconcerting randomness. Molima themselves live in a region dominated by 'matrilineal' descent, and I capitalise on Chowning's consistent scepticism about the utility of correlating types of descent with other features of social organisation, most recently expressed in her remark that Massim studies have tended to focus on unilineal groups as though maintaining them were the central concern of their members.

7 I have since read Bouquet's (in press) account of English kinship mediated by her teaching of British Social Anthropology in Portugal. The educated, middle-class 'English' taken as my reference point are defended as a category in Strathern (1992).

8 Note the construction. A discriminating axis that separates one domian from another reappears as a distinction internal to one or other domain. Fortes does this to Morgan's distinction between *societas* and *civitas*: modes of public life that discriminate whole evolutionary epochs are reconceptualised as spheres or domains of relations within a single society (see the critique in Mosko 1989).

9 Although the concept 'residual' was always used in a strictly relative sense, the impression is that cognatic ties were of secondary significance: however important non-lineal ties were for the individual person, they could not in this view carry sociocentric significance.

10 Fox (1967: 172), in reference to various types of cognatic kindred: 'Obviously the system of cognatic kindreds rings a bell for most readers as it resembles our own kinship system which is, however, unformalized and lacks named kindreds'. Conversely, Fortes (1969: 309, my emphasis): 'I regard it as now established that the elementary components of patrifiliation and matrifiliation, and hence of agnatic, enatic, and cognatic modes of reckoning kinship are, *like genes in the individual organism* invariably present in all familial systems.'

11 Freeman (1961: 200) lists those who, in the 1950s, were developing the term 'kindred' in the sense that European jurists had long used it (to refer to all of an individual's cognates).

12 Where persons are cut from persons (or relations from relations), as we might imagine a female agnate severed from her clan or donor

distinguished from recipient, then one position or perspective is substituted for another of comparable order. Thus Molima substitute the division of maternal and paternal kin at death for their combination in the living person. When persons die, they become reconstituted as siblings – their marriages, so to speak, undone and their children de-conceived. Now insofar as one set of relations (siblingship) substitutes for another (conjugality), it is also anticipated, and in that sense 'already there'. How different from the novelty with which English kinship (say) perceives the natural creation of individual persons and the social creation of relations!

PART III

Chapter 6 'Partners and Consumers', with the subtitle 'Making Relations Visible', was initially delivered at a conference convened by Natalie Davis, Rena Lederman and Ronald Sharp in 1990 on 'The Gift and its Transformations', National Humanities Center, North Carolina

Chapter 7 'A Partitioned Process' derives from a presentation to the second Melanesian Colloquium ('Embodiment and Sociality') held with Maurice Godelier, organised by James Weiner, at Manchester, 1991

Chapter 8 'Reproducing Anthropology', written in 1991, appears in *Contemporary Futures*, a monograph edited by Sandra Wallman for the Association of Social Anthropologists of the Commonwealth

CHAPTER 6

Partners and consumers

At the 1990 meetings of the British Association for the Advancement of Science, an experimental embryologist expounded an expert's view to a lay audience.[1] Johnson was concerned to demonstrate the continuity of biological process. A person's birth begins with primitive gametes laid down when one's parents were embryos in the grandparental womb. Subsequent development depends not only on genetic coding but on extra-genetic influences that operate on chromosomes from the start; these include stimulation from material enveloping the egg[2] as well as nutritive and other effects derived from placenta and uterus.

It was a powerful origin story (Franlin n.d.), especially in the context of current legislative decisions with respect to the Human Fertilisation and Embryology Act (1990). Here, however, the problem has been to formulate discontinuities between developmental phases. The House of Commons decided that research on human embryos is permissible up to 14 days, by which time, among other things, the pre-embryonic material is now discernibly divided into those cells that will form the future embryo−foetus and those that will form the placenta. The Secretary for Health was reported (*Guardian*, 24.4.1990) as saying that status as an individual could begin only at the stage where cells could be differentiated. Yet while biology appeared to provide an index,[3] the further problem of personhood raised the same notion of continuous process. Another member of the Commons pointed out: 'It is a very difficult matter to say at what stage do you have a citizen, a human being. At various stages fresh rights are acquired.' Rights can only be acquired of course, in this view, if there is an individual person to bear them (cf. Dunstan 1990: 6).

Here are experts informing lay persons (the BAAS talk), experts informing experts (the Secretary for Health is briefed on what the 14-day stage means), and lay persons (Members of Parliament) turning expert in making legislative decisions. An anthropologist might wish to bracket all of them lay insofar as they promote a common view of the person that, in his/her eyes, must have the status of a folk model. For the anthropological expert, 'person' is an analytic construct whose utility is evinced through cross-cultural comparison. One draws, as always, from one's culture of origin, but to be an expert in anthropology is to demonstrate simultaneously the cultural origins of one's analytic constructs and their cross-cultural applicability.

A person cannot in this sense be seen without the mediation of analysis. Yet those who discuss the potential personhood of the embryo implicitly contest such an appropriation of the concept. Visual representations of first the division of cells and then the human form as it takes shape regularly accompany not just talks designed to popularise the findings of science but attempts to make vivid the political issues at stake (cf. Petchesky 1987). Indeed, a flurry of fascination/repulsion was created by the Society for the Protection of Unborn Children which in April (while the Act as still in debate) sent all 650 MPs a life-sized model of a 20-week-old foetus. This parody of the ubiquitous free gift was intended to mobilise a parallel concern over the limit for legal abortions. The plastic foetus lifted out from a sectional womb,[4] and its message was clear. One can 'see' a (potential) person, and a person is known by its individuality. Individuality in turn means a naturally entire and free-standing entity: the claim was that at 20 weeks a foetus is a viable whole.

Between the anthropologist as expert and the lay person with his or her folk model lies more than an epistemological issue over what is usefully designated a 'person'; there is an ontological issue over the nature of the category. The anthropologist is dealing with a category that refers to certain analytical constructions. The laity may argue over what they see and what they call it but take for granted that the category refers to persons existing as visible and substantial entities. So while it may be hard to tell when a person begins, and while the law may have to define the stages at which rights accrue, it seems self-evident that the subject of these debates is a concrete human being. The anthropologist is not, of course, untouched by this cultural certitude.

Now for 'person' one could write 'gift'. That concept was drawn into anthropology from various domains of Western or

Euro-American discourse (economy, theology, and so forth) though its most notable proponents made out of the indigenous connotation of prestations voluntarily made an analytical category that also included the social fact of obligation. The point is that the concept of gift seemed readily applicable to self-evident and concrete 'gifts'. The term trailed a reassuring visualism. One could 'see' gift exchange because one could see the gifts, the things that people exchanged with one another. It also trailed a concern as Panoff (1970), Parry (1986) and others have noted, with individual autonomy (voluntarism) and interpersonal relations measured by degrees of interestedness (altruism).

As an anthropologist I am crippled, so to speak, by expertise – by the desire to appropriate the category 'gift' in a special way, insofar as those negotiations of relationships known as gift exchange in Melanesia have a character whose uniqueness I would be reluctant to relinquish. I say crippled to the extent that this position appears to set up barriers. Blind: I do not believe the evidence of my eyes, that one will recognise a gift when one sees it. Constricted: I cannot stride across the world map looking for gifts at all times and places. The wrong colour: monochrome rather than polychrome, for exhilarating as the company of other disciplines can be, I lose appropriative capability, feel very lay in the presence of other expertise. Other knowledge does not necessarily repair deficiencies in one's own – not something that concerns Melanesians, one should add, for they borrow from foreigners all the time, including the most intimate powers of reproduction.

Melanesians borrow origin stories, wealth and – as in the area I know best (Mount Hagen) – the expertise by which to organise their religion and their future. One clan takes from another its means of life. Indeed, exchanges surrounding the transfer of reproductive potential are intrinsic to the constitution of identity. From a clan's point of view, foreign wives are drawn to them by virtue of bride-wealth, and such items of wealth are themselves considered to have reproductive potential. Pigs create pigs and money creates money, as shell valuables also reproduce themselves, an idea given visible form in the iconography that developed with the influx of pearlshells into the Hagen area at the time of contact. Shells for circulation in gift exchange were mounted on resin boards vividly coloured with red ochre. The whole appeared a free-standing entity. But it was not an image of one. Rather than plastic moulding a visible homunculus, the child/embryo in its netbag/womb was indicated in the abstract by the curvature of the shell crescent, and the resin moulded a container around it.[5]

Personalised commodities?

In taking off from some of the expert discourse of Melanesian anthropology, I confine myself to certain issues in the under-standing of gifts, namely those concerned with reproduction and the life-cycle. It is arguable that all Melanesian gift exchanges are 'reproductive', but I make a more restricted point. The reason is to provide an approximation to the indigenous Euro-American understanding of gifts as 'transactions within a moral economy, which [make] possible the extended reproduction of social relations' (Cheal 1988: 19). My account ignores those aspects of the Melanesian gift that have seemed most strange to the twentieth-century Westerner (competition and the political striving for prestige), in order to focus on the apparently familiar (the celebration of kinship).

From the perspective of the Papua New Guinea Highlands, of the kind that Lederman (1986) has described for Mendi, I thus appear to privilege one nexus of gifting (kinship-based) over another (clan-based), or, more accurately, to evoke one type of sociality, for it is also arguable that each set of relations transforms the moral base of the other. But my interest is not in the relative moralities of exchanges (Parry and Bloch 1989). It is in whether Melanesian gifting can illuminate the very idea of there being part-societies ('moral economies') that 'typically consist of small worlds of personal relationships that are the emotional core of every individual's social experiences' (Cheal 1988: 15).

Whatever parallels might be useful for earlier European materials (e.g. Biagioli 1990), in the late twentieth century any understandings of such part-societies must in turn be put into their specific Euro-American context: consumer culture. Cheal himself goes on to give a consumerist definition of sociality. Everywhere (he says) people live out their lives in small worlds; the primitive (he says) because the societies were small, the modern because people 'prefer to inhabit intimate life worlds' (1988: 15).[6] Now recent anthropological discussion of the gift has turned, among other things, on the analytic advantage of distinguishing gift-based economies from commodity-based ones. Gregory (1982) has been notable here, and while his arguments explicated the contrast between gifts and commodities in terms of production, they have also opened up the question of consumption. In the formula he adopts, it is through consumption that things are drawn into the reproduction of persons, and reproduction can be understood as a process of personification. But consumption as a universal analytic is one thing. I take my own cue from the further fact that we live in a self-advertised 'consumer' culture.

A consumer culture is a culture, one might say, of personalisation. And to Euro-Americans, gift-giving seems a highly personalised form of transation. After all, it was the person in the gift that attracted anthropological attention to the concept in the first place. But whether useful parallels can be drawn between the personalisations of consumerisum and the personifications of Melanesian gift exchange remains to be seen.

Free-standing entities

The notorious individualism of Western culture has always seemed an abstraction of the state or of the market economy that lies athwart those concrete persons we recognise in interactions with others. No one is really an isolate. This was a point the embryologist wanted to get across, and for which he offered biological reasoning.

Johnson was concerned to demonstrate the influence of the environment in all stages of foetal development. Its significance for him lies in its contribution to the identity of the emergent individual: personal identity is the outcome not just of a unique genetic combination but of a unique history of continuous development which affects the way genetic factors themselves take effect. The organism is a finite and discrete entity; the process is continuous. Thus, he opined, an individual is always in interaction with its environment. This provoked a comment from the gynaecologist Modell who observed that, as far as the embryo is concerned, the environment is immediately the mother and the mother is *another person*. Among other things, the embryo undergoes the effects of the parents' changing perceptions of it.

The point slid by without much comment. What I see in that interchange is more than a dispute between experts, for it barely registered as a dispute. It epitomised the simultaneous delineation of a hegemonic model (of personhood) and the possibility of contesting it, somewhat parallel to the manner in which anthropologists have extricated the idea of gift from hegemonic understandings in Western culture in order to contest either the application of these under-standings to non-Western cultures or the dominance of the model in people's lives (cf. Josephides 1985). Modell's mild intervention sounded, in fact, almost like a version of critiques well rehearsed through the contested notion of rights in abortion debates. The right of the mother against the right of the child presents a contest of alternatives (cf. Ginsburg 1987). However, I wish to make a different kind of contest appear.

Johnson's idea of the individual person doubly defined by genetic programming and by environmental factors seems a solution to the old nature/nurture debate: we have, so to speak, put the individual back into its 'environment', in much the same way as social scientists are perpetually putting individuals back into 'society'. This is an individualism that gives full recognition to the context in which persons flourish, and we may read off from the image of the embryo an image of the individual person in a responsive, interactive and creative mode with the external world. Indeed, it is colloquial English to speak of an individual's 'relationship' to its environment as we do of an individual's 'relationship' to society.

But what a bizarre coupling! The whole person is held to be a substantial and visible entity. The environment, on the other hand, like society, is regularly construed as existing in the abstract, for it cannot be seen as a whole.[7] We may concretise the environment through examples of its parts, as uterus or as trees and mountains, as we may concretise society through referring to groups and insti-tutions. But there was more to Johnson's purpose. He wished to convey how it is potentially *everything* beyond the individual person that may influence that unique person and help make it what it is. The forces that continuously shape us are always, as he comments elsewhere, both genetic and epigenetic, and 'epigenetic' is the biologist's catch-all 'for everything else besides the genes' (1989: 39). I would add that this makes epigenetic factors of a different order from 'the genes' precisely in so far as 'everything else' is imagined, hypothetically and thus abstractly, as infinite. 'Myriad' is his word; the environment consists in this view of the sum of all the factors that might have an effect.

The view against which Johnson argues would hold that the whole and finite individual is determined largely by its genetic programming. But rather than context, perhaps we should see analogy between the conceptualisations here. Suppose the concept of the genetic programme were analogous to that of the individual, then the concept of epigenetic forces would appear analogous to that of environment/society. In turn, the relationship between genetic and epigenetic forces that Johnson postulates would be seen to miniaturise or replicate common-sense understandings of that between individual organism and an enveloping world. And the interest of Modell's remark would be in the way it cut across the analogies. For she displaced the image of a (finite, concrete) person contextualised by an (infinite, abstract) society/environment with another image: the exterior world imagined as another (finite, concrete) person.

She thus gave voice to a capability that also rests in English: of imagining a world that does not imagine such abstractions for itself, where sociality impinges in the presence of other persons. English speakers readily enough personify the agency of 'society' or even 'environment', though they would be hard put to think of these entities as persons. Yet that is exactly the way in which they might imagine that Melanesians imagine the world beyond themselves (e.g. Leenhardt 1979).[8] What contains the child is indeed 'another person', whether that other person is the mother, or the clan that nurtures its progeny, or the land that nurtures the clan and receives a fertilising counterpart in the burial of the placenta. This other person may be regarded as the cause or origin of the effective agency of those it contains (e.g. Wagner 1986b).

When Euro-Americans think of more than one person, they are faced with the disjunction of unique individuals and overcome this in the notion that individuals 'relate' to one another. What lie between them are relationships, so that society may be thought of as the totality of made relationships. That relationships are made further supposes that what are linked are persons as individual subjects or agents who engage in their making: 'interpersonal dependence is everywhere [!] the result of socially constructed ties between human agents' (Cheal 1988: 11). The idea of persons in the plural evokes, then, the image of the interactions between them, in turn the immediate social environment for any one of them.

It is because society is likened to an environment that it is possible for Euro-Americans to think of individual persons as relating not to other persons but to society as such, and to think of relations as after the fact of the individual's personhood rather than integral to it. Or so the folk model goes. Anthropologists, for their part, have captured the category of person to stand for subjects understood analytically in the context of social relations with others. In the particular way s/he looks to making 'society' visible (Miller 1987: 14), the anthropologist would be scandalised at the idea of a non-relational definition of persons.

The analytical necessity appears to have been given by just such societies as are found in Melanesia. Indeed, the anthropological experience may be that in such societies everything is relational. Certainly Melanesians constantly refer to the acts and thoughts of other persons. But if they seemingly situate themselves in a world full of what we call 'social relationships', such relationships do not link individuals. Rather, the fact of relating forms a background sociality to people's existence, out of which people work to make specific relationships appear (cf. J. Weiner 1988). Relations are thus integral to the person or, in Wagner's (1991) formulation, persons may be understood fractally: their dimensionality cannot be expressed in whole numbers. The fractal person is an entity with relationship integrally implied. Any scale of social activity mobilises the same dimensionality of person/relation.

There is no axiomatic evaluation of intimacy or closeness here. On the contrary, people work to create divisions between themselves. For in the activation of relations people make explicit what differentiates them (J. Weiner 1987). One may put it that it is the relationship between them that separates donor from recipient or mother from child. Persons are detached, not as individuals from the background of society or environment, but from other persons. However, detachment is never final, and the process is constantly recreated in people's dealings with one another. To thus be in a state of division with respect to others renders the Melanesian person dividual.

Persons are not conceptualised, therefore, as free-standing. A Hagen clan is composed of its agnates and those foreigners detached from other clans who will give birth to its children; a woman contains the child that grows through the acts of a man; shells are mounted on the breast. One person may 'carry' another, as the origin or cause of its existence and acts. An implicate field of persons is thus imagined in the division or dispersal of bodies or body parts (Mimica 1988; Gillison 1991). From their viewpoint,

Euro-Americans cannot readily think of bodies and body parts as the substance of people's interactions. They can imagine objects flowing between persons 'as though' they 'symbolised' body parts, but for them to discover that a shell is like a foetus in a womb is simply to uncover an image, a metaphorical statement about (say) fertility. So let me return to the embryologist's address and to a moment when he seemed at a loss for a metaphor.

During his presentation, Johnson flashed on the screen a picture of twin babies with their common placenta between them. The three were genetically identical, he briefly observed. Three what? One may fill in the silence, that of course they were not three persons, for only the twins, not the placenta, would grow into autonomous subjects. The placenta is regarded as a source of support, at once part of the foetus and part of the foetus's environment, yet only through detachment from it is the individual person made;[9] the picture included the cut cords and the scissors that cut them. Not at all how the Melanesian 'Are 'Are of Malaita in the Solomon Islands would see it. There the placenta both remains part of the person and, in becoming detached at birth, is treated as another person. Detachment is conceptualised as a separation of (dividual) persons from one another.

De Coppet (1985) describes how the placenta is buried in ancestral land, linking the living person to a network of ancestral funeral sites and returning to source two vital parts of personal substance. It is planted like a dead taro that has lost its living stem (the baby); taro denotes 'body'. The 'Are 'Are placenta is also referred to as the baby's pig, an allusion to animate 'breath'. (What the placenta lacks is a third part, the ancestral 'image' that adults assume when they die naturally, that is, are killed by their own ancestors; the un-imaged placenta is buried somewhat after the manner of an un-imaged murder victim). Pig and taro assure the vitality of the living child; it is also expected that scavenging pigs will eat the buried placenta and that taro will grow there. The land that nourishes the child is also constituted of what constitutes the living person and is a cause of its life. 'Are 'Are personify the land, territorialise the person. When one understands how the land owns people, de Coppet was told,[10] one can understand how people own land.

This relationship to the land is not quite the same as the English-speaking conceptualisation of a (concrete) person's relationship to the (abstract) environment/society. For the 'Are 'Are person (land) thereby *enters into an exchange* with the land (person). If your placenta has been buried, 'it proves that, in return for your life, through the land, you have given back the share of "body" and "breath" which must rejoin the universal circulation' (de Coppet 1985: 87).

It is for such a world as this, where persons' actions always seem to be caused by or elicited by other 'persons', that the borrowed concept of the gift captures what a Westerner would sense as a pervasive sociality. It seems just the formula to emphasise the personal nature of interpersonal relations. Perhaps that is because in turn gifts typify a sector of Western culture which seemingly parallels the pervasive sociality of Melanesian life: the close inter-personal relations of kinship and friendship. Here one gives and takes on an intimate basis. Yet the appearance of similarity is, inevitably, misleading. Euro-American intimacy is signalled by two constructs peculiar to it, altruism and voluntarism.

Altruism: donors and partners

Advances in reproductive medicine that have highlighted artificial mechanisms to assist procreation have also heightened certain Western perceptions of the interaction between procreating partners. Thus in the context of discussing artificial insemination by donor, Sissa recalls the assumption 'that semen is donated, the uterus only loaned' (1989: 133; cf. Stolcke 1986).[11] That paternity should in addition be thought a matter of opinion, maternity a matter of fact, turns not on the certainty about donation but on certainty about social identity. It is because semen has the appearance of a (visible) detachable bodily substance that it seems alienable. Because it is alienable, its source may be in doubt. Both the substantial nature of semen and the asymmetry of the relationship between semen and uterus (individual and environment) present an inverse of the supposition found in Aristotle, that semen provided form and maternal blood the substance of the child. The potency of semen in this ancient view was that it was efficacious in the way a craftsman's activities were efficacious; it had an activating force on female blood but did not contribute particles of matter to the embryo. The movement of the male body, the act of donation, constituted the male part in procreation.[12]

Sissa draws the inevitable parallel with the Trobriands, between the multiple fathering made possible by donor insemination (DI) and the fact (as she puts it) that the Trobriand child has two fathers, one whose semen moulds somatic identity and one (the mother's brother) who defines the kin group to which the child belongs. Yet the parallel is a poor one, since the social identity of the Trobriand father is integral to his somatic role, whereas in the case of DI knowing the father's identity is both optional and after the fact of the donation. Donation linking a person to a source of genetic endowment does not necessarily link the person to another person. Indeed, twentieth-century people who talk of semen 'donation' treat it as a substance that will fertilise the maternal egg *whether or not* its identity is known. This is the crux. Semen is potentially alienable (from the body), I suggest, because of the possibility of its being produced without being elicited by another person. This is, in turn, a general conceptual possibility, regardless of whether or not DI is at issue, captured in its visual representation as a detachable substance.[13] DI adds the further conceptual possibility, that conception need not be accompanied by bodily movement; movement is only required to produce the semen. Sissa points out that Aristotle's emphasis on the transcendent and non-substantial aspect of the semen led him to assert it could never be frozen, whereas twentieth-century people keep frozen specimens in banks for future use.

Nonetheless, the new reproductive technologies have repaired some of the asymmetry, for it would seem that 'egg donation' has passed into the lay imagination as a process analogous to semen donation.[14] Anonymity may or may not be preserved. In the case of maternal surrogacy, however, a partnership of a kind has to be set up between the commissioning couple and the surrogate mother. People talk crudely of womb-renting, or more delicately of the gift of life.[15]

Donation is here conceptualised in two ways. On the one hand it may simply involve an act of bodily emission intended for an anonymous recipient; on the other hand it may involve a relationship between donors and recipients as partners in a single enterprise. This corresponds to the double conceptualisation of sociality in consumer culture, as much a matter of an individual's relationship to society in the abstract as of interaction between concrete persons.

The terminology of donation and gift is seeminly encouraged by clinical and other experts by virtue of this double evocatory power. It evokes the charitable altruism of blood and organ donors;

it also evokes the intimate altruism of transactions that typify personal relations outside the market. (1) Organ donors can give anonymously because human organs are regarded as anonymous: kidneys differ in physical condition rather than social identity (however, see Abrahams 1990).[16] Such organs or materials as can be excised or secreted from the body become free-standing entities. So although semen carries formative genetic material that will contribute to a person's identity, it is also possible to think of contributing one's part to a general supply. Donation here carries connotations of the charitable gesture, the personal sacrifice for the public good, a gift to society. (2) Alternatively, sometimes in the case of egg donation and certainly of willingness to carry a child, altruism may be embedded in specific relations. A partnership is created between donor and recipient. An egg donated from a close relative can thus be regarded as belonging to a relationship that already exists, an expression of love. The carrying mother, related or not, is regarded as sacrificing comfort and ease in order to enable others to have children; because of the nature of her labour, and the attempt to protect such acts from commercial exploitation, as in the case of charity the language of gift-giving becomes the language of altruism.

But do these gestures and does this language constitute a gift economy?

Cheal (1988) has argued exactly this in examining the nexus of present-giving among friends and relatives, as at Christmas and birthdays, in suburban Canada. Gifts indicate community member-ship (the reproduction of social status) as well as relations of intimacy. In either case, they symbolise the central values of a 'love culture', he argues, whether the love is generally or specifically directed. We encounter here the same double: gifts for society and gifts for persons. Cheal introduces a further distinction between the immediate society of the moral economy (his 'small world', the real community) and the further society of the political economy. Gifts make gestures of altruism within, it would seem, the near society, whereas the far society is seen as a realm of commerce. It is in their immediate circles that persons 'make' relationships as they 'make' love, and community-giving is a diffuse, impersonal version of intimacy-giving.

While I would dispute neither the evocation of emotions and (society-near) relational behaviour among friends and relatives nor the way this mobilises conventions distinct from those that regulate other (society-far) areas of life, I add one comment: *the circulation of gifts does not create distinct kinds of persons.* 'Gifts' (presents) are free-standing entities just like commodities, 'alienable', as Cheal says. Indeed the person who purchases a present to give to a friend simply puts in reverse the same process which makes it possible for him/her to donate body substance to a blood bank, cadaver to science. An anonymously produced object becomes part of a store on which others draw. Preserving the social anonymity of market goods is, of course, fundamental to the supposition that goods are available for all. That such goods can be appropriated by the consumer and fashioned to the ends of personal identity (Miller 1987, 1988) – the wrapped present, the exhibited taste – is part of the cultural interpretation of consumption as consumerism.[17]

While they may express personal identity, *goods do not have to be made into gifts* in order to do so. Gifts between persons can make statements about relationships, yet a relationship is not necessary to the creation of identity. The analogy with reproductive process is evident: genetic identity does not imply a social relationship.

As I understand it, what Euro-Americans call gifts in late-twentieth-century consumer culture, whether body substance or merchandise, are regarded as extensions of the self insofar as they carry the expression of sentiments. Sentiments are commonly expressed toward other persons, but they may equally well be directed to abstract entities such as 'society'. For sentiments emanate outwards from the person, *whether or not they are 'received' by specific others.* They thus appear as the person would like to appear, autonomous, charitable. Sentiment is supposed to have positive connotations in the same way as near relations are supposed to be benign, and presents carry positive overtones of sociability and affection. Hence Cheal's closeted language of community and intimacy.

Indeed, the kinds of presents Cheal describes are like the 'goods' of classical economy: objects of desire. It is individuals, he observes, who give and receive goods and who reproduce their relations with others, though they do so, I would add, from their own vantage point (of desire). Cheal (1988: 10) himself offers a comparison; he takes the free disposition of items as distinguishing the gift in the moral economy of suburban Canada from those reciprocities allegedly described by Gregory (1982) that put people into a state of bondage (his term, not Gregory's). It is the alienability of the former that confers freedom. The sentiment such items express springs from within the individual person, and it is the flow of sentiment (the ideology of love) that makes relationships. As a consequence, Euro-American gift-giving really only works as a sign of personal commitment if it is also a sign of benign feeling. Benign feeling in turn is presented as an attribute of the small-scale, with its dialectic of intimacy and community. This confident equation of the small-scale with the interpersonal is, to say the least, an interesting cultural comment on the dimensions of persons.

Where the cycling of gifts among kin effects the procreation and regeneration of relationships, this can comprise activity of a cosmic order. Consider the Melanesian Sabarl on the eastern tip of the Massim archipelago (Battaglia 1990). Not only is this tiny dialect group of fewer than a thousand people able to account for the beginning of time, their gift exchanges are of universal dimensions. No part-societies here: the entire system of production, distribution and consumption is a process of personification 'that converts food and objects and people into other people' (1990: 191, emphasis removed). And society does not exist apart from other people; rather, persons are of global dimensions, sociality integral to them. This is made evident by their parentage. A person is forever a dependant with respect to his or her father's clan, with whom he/she is involved in a lifetime of exchanges. Dependency is conceptualised in terms of specific relations: a member of the father's clan acts as a designated 'father' to the eternal 'child' whom he 'feeds', an activity that lasts from conception till burial when it must be stopped (Battaglia 1985). In this matrilineal society, paternal kin are keepers of mortality and the father's donations have effect (only) for as long as the child lives. This is no more nor less 'bondage' than one might say one is a slave to life or, in Aristotle's terms, a victim of paternal motility.

The partner in such exchanges is always another and specific person. Gifts are never free-standing: they have value because they are attached to one social source ('father') in being destined for another ('child') and, whether they originate in labour or in other transactions, carry identity. Yet when all such encounters are interpersonal encounters, they convey no special connotations of intimacy. Nor of altruism as a source of benign feeling.

The Western notion of persons being contained by their environment/society is indeed significant here, though not quite for

Johnson's reasons. It enables Euro-Americans to think of the gift as altruistic by the conceivable analogy of a gesture towards exactly such abstract entities.[18] Altruistic gestures toward other persons are invariably tempered by the after-effect of realising that one's own self-interest must be bound up somewhere, if only in maintaining one's (social) environment. Conversely, it is possible to think of gifts as voluntarily given despite social pressure and obligation precisely because they conventionally typify those relations that are made through the spontaneous emission of emotions.

Voluntarism: recipients and consumers

Consumer culture, it would seem, springs from the perpetual emanations of desire held to radiate from each individual person. This well-spring is like the bottomless pit of need that Euro-Americans are also supposed to suffer, such as the celebrated biological need for women to have children – a 'drive to reproduce' (quoted in Stanworth 1987: 15). In meeting need and desire, the individual person expresses the essential self. A rhetoric of accumulation is thus bound to the voluntarism of individual effort. One might remark that the constant necessity for the individual to implement his or her subjectivity has its own coercive force.

If there is a similarity between the coercions of gift-giving in Melanesia and late-twentieth-century consumerism, then we may indeed find its echo in the desire/drive/need for the individual to act as a free agent. With two differences. First, that on the Melanesian side the need is located not in the agent but in those 'other persons' who cause the agent to act. Second, that Melanesian accumulation is tempered by the fact that acts, like relations, work to substitutive effect. Relations are not perpetually 'made'. Rather, relations are either made to appear or appear in their making; every new relationship displaces a former one. Each gift is a substitution for a previous gift. One extracts from another what one has had extracted from oneself. Thus de Coppet points to the chain of transformations that constitute the common task on which 'Are 'Are society is based. As endless process of perpetual dissolution by which 'objects, animals, persons, or elements of persons' (1981: 201) change continuous decay into life.

As elsewhere in Austronesian-speaking Melanesia (Damon and Wagner 1989), a death divides survivors into mourners (feast givers) and workers (who bury the deceased and are feasted).* In 'Are 'Are each side makes a pile of food, topped with money, which reconstitutes the dead person. Not only do both piles incorporate foot items from the other, the two piles are then exchanged. They replace the deceased with a composition both of the relations once integral to him or her, and of his or her basic elements: 'body' (taro and coconut), 'breath' (pork) and 'image' (money). These replacements enable the deceased's body/breath to be consumed, and later themselves replaced by a further display composed entirely of money. First the workers take charge of it, then reassemble it for the mourners (the deceased's family) to dispose of; the latter return all the wealth received in the course of the funeral and thereby complete the final element, the ancestor's image (1981: 188). The new ancestor is now accessible to his living descendants.

De Coppet refers to 'replacement' rather than substitution (1981: 202, n. 17), which for him carries too many resonances of displacing one individual object by another. Yet, as we have seen, what are also replaced are not just the elements that compose an individual but the relationships of which the person is composed. A relationship is 'replaced' through the substitution of a counterpart. The point is explicit in Battaglia's account of Sabarl mortuary ritual, where the actions of mourning and burial mobilise the respective maternal and paternal kin of the deceased. That person is visibly reconstituted in the assembling of funeral foods (sago pudding) and wealth (axe blades), semen and bones being simultaneously returned by maternal kin to the paternal.

These are gifts of life. Life is given in the necessity to consume the deceased as a physical presence and thus release the future – the ancestor to future descendants – from present relationships. As a consequence, the relations that composed and supported the deceased must be made finally visible. Most importantly, in the course of the funeral feasts, relations between maternal and paternal kin appear in the division between donors and recipients. The 'father' makes a final prestation of axe blades; maternal kin then substitute for these blades of their own and hand back the items with increment. But more than this. Food and valuables are composed into an image of the deceased before being given to the paternal kin. The Sabarl

* The Trobriand Islanders and Molima mentioned in Chapter 5, as well as the North Mekeo drawn upon in Chapter 4, are Austronesian-speakers.

deceased is thus rendered into a form at once visible (in the abstract) and dissoluble (in its substance): its components can be consumed or dissipated. 'People consume other people' (Battaglia 1990: 190). The dead die because the link between persons out of which the person was born is dissolved.

Insofar as one might imagine elements of this exchange sequence as involving the transfer of gifts, the obligation to receive cannot be reduced to the enactment of any one particular exchange. For the person to die, relationships must be undone. And once the person has died, paternal kin on Sabarl can no more avoid being the recipients of funeral gifts than the maternal body in Western discourse can avoid bearing a child.

Sabarl recipients are also consumers: that is, they turn these things (food, valuables) into their own bodies (to be eaten, distributed). Maternal kin dissipate the composed body in order to recompose anew. Similarly de Coppet suggests that 'Are 'Are life is dominated by the fact that it is one's own kin who have the ultimate right to consume one, body and breath being thereby absorbed back into body and breath to be available for future generations. The capacity to consume is thus the capacity to substitute future relations for past ones. It depends on a double receptivity – to reabsorb parts of oneself and to be open to the (body) parts of others. The difference between death and life is the absence or presence of such relationships with 'other' persons.

The Melanesian recipient of a gift who puts wealth into the recesses of a house, as a clan contains the external sources of its fertility within, is literally consuming the gift. But the vitalising power of the gift lies in the fact that it derives from an exogenous source. One attaches and contains the parts of specific others, for the process of attachment and detachment is the motility that signals life. Actions are registered (fractually) in the actions of other persons, each person's acts being thereby replaced, reconstituted, in new and even foreign persons/forms. Thus is the living person personified.

By contrast, the latter-day Euro-American consumer draws from an impersonal domain, such as the market, goods that, in being turned into expressions of self-identity, become personalised. The exercise of choice is crucial; choice creates consumption as a subjective act. To evince subjectivity is to evince life. One may even appear to exercise 'more' subjectivity in some situations/relationships than in others. This rather bizarre notion – that ideally one ought always to act as a subject but cannot always do so — is symbolised in the special domain of interpersonal relations.

The Euro-American person is presented, then, as a potentially free-standing and whole entity (an individual subject or agent) contained within an abstract impersonal matrix which may include other persons but also includes other things as its context (environment/society). And this is the image of the consumer. Consumer choice is thinkable, I would suggest, precisely insofar as 'everything else' is held to lie beyond the foetus/embryo/person: *anything consumed by that person comes from the outside,* whether or not the source is other persons. For generative power lies in the individual person's own desire for experience. Desire and experience: the principal dimensions of the consumer's relationship with his/her environment. And the field is infinite; it consists of the sum of all the possibilities that may be sampled. Satisfied from without, the impetus is held to spring from within.[19] While individual desires may be stimulated by the outside world — advertising, marketing and so forth — that in turn is supposed to be oriented to the consumer's wants.

Whereas the Melanesian capacity to receive has to be nurtured in and elicited from a partner, sometimes to the point of coercion, the twentieth-century consumer is depicted as having infinite appetite. Above all, the consumer is a consumer of experience and thus of him-/herself. Perhaps it is against the compulsion of appetite, the coercion of having to choose, the prescriptiveness of subjective self-reference, that the possibility of unbidden goods and unanticipated experiences presents itself as exotic. The 'free gift'.

* * *

My assertions have no doubt resisted certain common-sense formulations (one cannot see a gift) only to substitute others (we know what a consumer is). And to suggest that the issues which the concept of the gift trails through anthropological accounts — a relational view of the person, altruism, voluntarism — have to be understood in terms of its culture of origin is hardly original. But perhaps the particular substitution I mention here has interest. Given the part that so-called gift exchange plays in the reproduction of persons in Melanesia, it was not inapposite to consider the new language of gifting that accompanies the propagation of late-twentieth-century reproductive technologies. There we discover the Euro-American person as a free-standing entity interacting with its environment, a figure missing from the twentieth-century Melanesian pantheon. The first question to ask, then, is what kind of person the Melanesian gift reproduces.

The double orientation of gifts in consumer culture presupposes two kinds of relationships: an individual person's interpersonal relations with others and an individual person's relations with society. Melanesian gifts on the other hand presuppose two kinds of persons, partners divided by their transaction: paternal from maternal kin, foetus from placenta, clansmen from the ground they cultivate, descendants from ancestors. Gifts may come from an outside source, but that source is hardly imagined as beyond persons in the way the talents and the riches of the world seemingly come from God in Davis's (n.d.) sixteenth-century France.[20] For even where the other person is imagined as a deity or spirit or as the very land itself, the Melanesian act of giving that divides recipient from donor presupposes a partnering of finite identities. By contrast, the gift capable of extending a personalised self into a potentially infinite universe turns the person into a potential recipient of everything.

Late-twentieth-century and Euro-American, the embryo visualised as a homunculus is a consumer in the making. For the consumer actualises his or her relationship with society/the environment in its own body process. This prompts a second question: whether gift-giving in a consumer culture contests the coercive nature of this relationship or is another example of it.

Notes

1 See also Johnson 1989. The BAAS meetings are intended to present scientific investigations and discoveries to the public. The debate, *Human Embryo Research: What Are the Issues?*, was organised by the Ciba Foundation.

2 The early conceptus is dependent on the developmental history of the egg in the mother, which provides 'a mature physical and biochemical entity within which the whole complex process' of early development operates (Johnson 1989: 40), an interaction quite distinct from the egg's genetic contribution to the conceptus.

3 To the lay person. To the embryologist, 'Biology does not tell us that a line should or should not be drawn' (Johnson 1989: 41); it is the job of legislation to draw the lines.

4 The foetus was entire (a homunculus), but its cord was severed, and the womb was in half-section with the placenta visibly sectioned as well. The severed cord was painted in such a way as to invite horror at the tearing away of the foetus; but the womb itself was 'severed' for no other purpose, it would seem, than to have it provide a convenient cup for the model of the foetus. A simulated horror.

5 The shell is both procreative and procreated. This point was stimulated by two then unpublished papers in which Jeffrey Clark analysed the remarkable iconography of Wiru pearlshells; see Clark 1991. Goldlip pearlshells were prized but scarce before European contact. Young children are carried by their mothers in looped 'string' bags, known by the same term as that for the womb.

6 In the 1990s, life-world-style life worlds are already passé, if one is to believe upmarket consumer experts. I refer to the concept of the personalised market here. 'If the modern world is based on the notion of an endless repetition of a few products, then its successor is based on the idea of short-runs and the targeting of many, different, products' (Jencks and Keswick 1987: 48–9), though, as Jencks observes, individual tastes are not as variable as the potential production of variety.

7 I read this off from Johnson's presentation of the epigenetic factors. These were indicated in highly generalised terms by contrast with the specific representation of the foetus/person. No doubt his professional view is more sophisticated than the image I have derived from his talk (an organism as a free-standing entity within an environment to which it 'adapts'), but for a critique of similar perceptions as they have informed the concept of culture in anthropology, see Ingold (n.d.).

8 For non-Melanesian depictions of the world imagined as a plurality of bodies and of the body containing a plurality of worlds, see the chapters by Malamoud and Lévi in Feher *et al.* (1989).

9 Morgan (1989) observes that in the United States it is generally thought that the neonate becomes a person with the cutting of the umbilical cord.

10 My interpretation of the sequence of statements made to de Coppet by the paramount chief Eerehau.

11 The term 'semen' may be used either as the vehicle that carries sperm or as an alternative for sperm itself. It is sperm donation that is strictly at issue here.

12 Rather in the way that gifts of money in 'Are 'Are encompass, transcend and differentiate the three components of the person (body, breath and image) (de Coppet 1981, 1985), so Aristotelian semen is the vehicle for the three 'principles', soul, form and movement (Sissa 1989: 136).

13 However, its alienability is a contested point. A recent study by Jeanette Edwards (pers. comm.) points to diverse views on men's part about the extent to which semen is or is not felt to be disposable in the way body organs potentially are.

14 The relative complexities of the techniques render the physical operations quite different (Price 1989: 46–7). While artificial semen donation is a 200-year-old practice, scientific papers about pregnancies from donated oocytes did not appear in professional journals until 1983–4 (Frances Price, pers. comm.).

15 A phrase applied to interventionist medicine in general. In a world of punning acronyms, it is no accident that GIFT should occur, though for a process (gamete intra-fallopian transfer) that need involve no 'donation' from outside sources.

16 Ties are occasionally established between the relatives of organ donors and the recipients. Abrahams, drawing on analogies with gift-giving, explores both what is new and what is old in the identities set up by organ transplant; 'racial' origin remains an uninvited guest at the debate.

17 For non-consumerist appropriations, I cite two examples. One is Werbner's (1990) remarkable account of 'capital, gifts and offerings among British Pakistanis'; the other Yang's (1989) critique of 'second-economy' arguments in relation to gifts and the state redistributive economy in contemporary China.

18 Parry arguing on this point also reinstates Mauss's purpose in *The Gift* as demonstrating just how we ever came to contrast interested and disinterested gifts. 'So while Mauss is generally represented as telling us how in fact the gift is never free, what I think he is really telling us is how we have acquired a theory that it should be' (1986: 458, emphasis omitted). I merely point here to the further coercions of choice in the consumer world of compulsory subjectivity.

19 I am compressing several arguments and contested positions here, and do not specify where the view is held. It alludes but does not do justice to Miller's (1987) reading of consumption as symbolic labour (the consumer recontextualises the commodity and objectifies it afresh as a source of inalienable value).

20 For a Melanesian Christian counterpart, see Gregory (1980).

CHAPTER 7

A partitioned process

By and large a biological approach to the beginnings of life is rooted in gradualism ... The same is true in the development of individual lives. They begin with chemistry and they reach their fulfilment in mystery ... Biologically speaking we are looking at a continuous process.
(John Habgood, Archbishop of York, House of Lords, Official Record, 7 December 1989, col. 1020)

The Archbishop of York was addressing the House of Lords on the development of human life. The context was the second reading of the then Human Fertilisation and Embryology Bill, where debate was directed largely towards the question of embryo research. The government's proposal included a recommendation about the time limit within which research would be allowed.* Those in favour were concerned to establish the validity of a limit through developmental criteria; opponents to the actual idea of research included those for whom the embryo's potential was unaffected by stage of development.

A consensus underlying the debate was that experimentation on human beings was unethical. The proponents of research were concerned, therefore, to establish a divide in time which would correspond to a divide in the identity of the emergent embryo. Before a certain point one would be dealing with relatively undifferentiated matter; after a certain point the first conditions for a potential individual could be recognised and one could start talking of the origins of a future human being. The Archbishop argued that it was a mistake to suppose that human beings came into existence at conception and all that happened thereafter was that they grew. Biological gradualism revealed a process that was continuous, as was also true of (he said) evolution, and a process that had one very important characteristic. It concerned not just growth but development:[1] 'early embryos are not miniature babies. What is lacking in that perception

---

* The House of Commons decision was still in the future.

is any understanding of how, biologically speaking, the process of development creates the person' (House of Lords, Official Record, 7 December 1989, col. 1021). He then added that the biological view could be backed by a theological understanding of creation as continuous – 'God continuously calling personal being into existence'.

Because the process is regarded as continuous, the movement from one state of being (early embryo) to another (person) appears as an uninterrupted flow. His point, however, was that the flow is not simply one of magnification. As the material develops it becomes more complex, and in this view personhood is a function of a certain stage of complexity. The process of becoming more complex is continuous, then, but degree of complexity means that the final entity has different characteristics from its precursor. At several moments in the debate to which Habgood contributed, the early embryo was described in terms of its primitive cellular formation. As a former experimental biologist observed, at one stage in our lives all of us were just made up of a few cells.

The House considered many issues; let me indicate the interest that lies in these particular formulations.

The problem of development

Development not only describes movement from one condition to another – from early embryo to person, as it was put. It also implies that certain original conditions continue to be relevant (a human being continues to be made up of cells) even though those conditions do not exhaust the description of the entire being (a person is more than cells). Here the second entity is imagined as of a different order from the first and as thus encompassing what is also of a different order from itself. A similar asymmetric relationship inheres in the way language itself is partitioned.

'What is happening embryologically', the Archbishop said on a later occasion (quoted in Morgan and Lee 1991: 71, my emphasis), 'is the creation of *persons* through a process, which although it begins with genetic union, is not simply about a union of genes but also depends on a certain *cellular* identity'.[2] It is one, he added, 'which only becomes apparent at the time of the appearance of the primitive streak [the precursor of body tissue]'. The speaker in effect moves between semantic domains – from the language of the cultural definition of a social entity (person) to the language of natural, biologically defined, material (cell). This was, I believe, a general characteristic of the embryo debate. A further partition emerges in the perception of what was at issue. No one – in this context – disputed the description of early cellular formation; its factual basis was taken for granted. There was dispute about how its status should be interpreted; this was understood as the interpretation *of* the facts.[3]

An asymmetry appears in both instances, at least insofar as one kind of knowledge is regarded as dependent on or as the subject of another kind of knowledge. The one may also appear as the ground of the other, or as encompassing of it.

Where interpretation (at which point in the process one can talk of a human being or person) is held to depend on a prior fact (the state of cellular formation), then it would seem that the act of interpretation itself only 'becomes' appropriate at a certain point in describing the developmental process. Degree of (natural) complexity invites degree of (social) interpretation. Parliament was having to grapple with scientific information about embryology and at the same time come to a decision for legislative purposes. Each piece of information might clarify the last, but the addition of information also increased the complexity of the issues. And the relationship between facts and the interpretation of them was a serious one. Intervention to determine the point beyond which developing embryonic material could no longer be a suitable subject for experiment would affect the kind of scientific information available to future generations.

What was being debated was thus to some extent paralleled in the fact of debate itself. The description of the manner in which biologically defined material 'becomes' a human person was a particular issue for those promoting the viewpoint of biological continuity; but they drew on a generally shared precept. The question was when one can recognise in a natural form the presence of a social one. In posing the very question, speakers drew on natural facts to ground their interpretations; at the same time they interpreted facts to ground their viewpoints. Facts thereby became simultaneously the ground for argument and the subject of interpretation. This is indeed a common facility of the language they were using. Either fact or interpretation can operate in an encompassing (grounding) mode, that is, either can seem the origin of the distinction between them. And either can appear simple or complex in relation to the other. For example, 'interpretation' understood *as* the relationship between fact and interpretation appears as a complex interaction in that the more complex the observer's interpretative skills, the more complex the facts appear; by contrast the 'facts' of biological development may be held to show a (simple) progression from a simple to a complex state. Following this example, we might say that the person contains within itself the distinction between cell and person; the cell does not. But one may equally well see the facts as the source of complexity, and interpretation as derivative.

However, it is not the encompassing character of the terms I wish to pursue here. I shall discuss an asymmetry, but it is one contained in a particular notion of development or process itself.

This rests in the way a cumulative sequence can be presented as a matter of form building on form and that itself as a kind of addition. As the Archbishop said in reference to the biology of human development, 'one might call it a value-added process' (House of Lords, Official Record, 7 December 1989, col. 1020). Similarly, when it is acknowledged that because people have viewpoints facts will be interpreted in particular ways, that process is regarded as adding social and cultural complexity to an original understanding of the facts themselves. And when ethical discussions of personhood are felt to lie within the province of the House, but outside the province of embryology [see n. 3, Chapter 6], then ethical issues appear in addition to the natural ones.

In this world-view, what is added also brings about a modification of the original – and renders the relationship between the terms asymmetrical. Process is cumulative: the addition is not of equal parts, a simple doubling of the original, but of new features that augment or supplement it. The appearance of the primitive streak gives a new identity to the embryonic cells. But when each feature is also an element regarded as deriving from a domain of phenomena or expertise with its own conventions and character, the addition remains visible. It retains an irreducible character, one that rests on a prior differentiation or partitioning in the objects of knowledge. Ethical considerations, for instance, can be no more than grafted on to the understanding of scientific information. The result is a kind of conceptual hybrid – the character of one entity (biological information about human cells) modified by the character of another (ethical debate about the treatment of persons).

It follows that, by virtue of retaining their distinct character, elements so combined may also be prised apart or partitioned again.

The reverse of addition is subtraction. Despite their different positions, speakers in the House of Lords debate seemingly shared the premise that there was a difference between the natural facts of biological process and the human meanings put on them. The two were kept apart, as though one could indeed be subtracted from the other. While scientific language was as much a human construction as the language of ethics, in this view, the aim of scientific language was factual description rather than the promotion of an opinion or point of conscience.

Yet here the parallel I have been drawing between the parliamentary debate and the development of the embryo being discussed seems to falter. After all, under normal conditions the cumulative process of human development and complexification cannot be partitioned: that is, one cannot subsequently 'subtract' the cells from the person, prise them apart. However, one most certainly can in the imagination (and more, as we shall see), and most certainly in the language of the imagination. That is in any case what we understand as analysis.

Like developing cells, language has a constant potential for increasing differentiation although, unlike them, can always be put into reverse. This potential means that the divisive, fragmenting effects of language use have to be overcome in the very effort to delineate developmental process as cumulative and continuous. But the problem for the proponents of gradualism doubled back on itself. For they could not use identical terms for both beginning and end of the process since that would cede the arguments of those who claimed human beings were there from the start. They had to retain a terminological distinction. At least, this is a problem for which I surmise one most interesting solution was offered. It turned on the representation of complexity itself. In brief, the notion that complexity is a matter of degree (a view which suggests discontinuity between stages and allows a distinction of terms) could be subsumed under the idea that any one stage is the outcome of a process of complexification (a continuous sequence to be rendered as a single concept).

At one point in the debate, and in a single superb stroke, Habgood momentarily released prior interpretations from their dependence on the facts and neutralised the question of the degree of development by turning the whole process of complexification into the prior fact of life that needed understanding. He did so by introducing a metaphor.

The metaphor was patently artificial in the circumstances, but it was offered as an 'as if' way of imagining real-life developmental process. Here was the solution. The metaphor occupied the obvious place of a constructed act of interpretation. Its subject, how complex entities (such as persons) develop from simple ones (such as an embryonic cellular mass), occupied the place of natural fact. Developmental process thus appeared as a self-contained domain insofar as it required interpretation. My surmise is that assisting interpretation by so partitioning off this 'natural' domain through the artificiality of the metaphor had the effect of glossing over existing partitions between (natural) fact and (social) interpretation. The flow from 'cell' to 'person', like the flow from 'scientific information' to 'legislative decision', could be rendered continuous.

The metaphor so brilliantly summoned was an artificial graft, one that bore no intrinsic relationship to the subject of embryo development. But it added a measure of understanding. For the metaphor was held to illuminate the naturalness of complexity itself. Indeed, it led to an unfolding analogy for how one might think about the relationship between different stages in embryo development; the same analogy also illuminated the parliamentarians' developing understanding of the issues involved. The former intention was explicit in the Archbishop's statement; the latter I have added by way of my own interpretation. I do so in order to comment on the role of such analogies in the imagining of relationships.

Mandelbrot in the House of Lords

An entire passage from the statement that the Archbishop of York made to the House of Lords is itself reproduced by Morgan and Lee 'as a metaphor [which could serve] not just for embryonic existence and human life but for the whole of the moral debates which these issues engendered' (1991: 72). It contains the Archbishop's own metaphor, that of the Mandelbrot set. He unfolds it as an analogy for processual relationships.

> Perhaps I can make the significance of this a little more clear by giving your Lordship an analogy. Exactly 10 years ago a mathematician called Mandelbrot first discovered what is now called the Mandelbrot set. It is a set of points which can be mapped out as a computer graphic to form the most amazing, beautiful and complex structure that it is possible to imagine. It is a picture of literally infinite depth. If one magnifies the

details of any part of the picture, one finds that in them are whole worlds of further detail which are always beautiful, which never repeat themselves and which always reveal more and more detail, on and on, *ad infinitum.*

How is the Mandelbrot set made? It is made by the use of an absurdly simple equation with only three terms. The secret lies in the process. It is a process whereby the answer to one use of the equation becomes the starting point for the next. In other words, it is a cumulative process, just like evolution in which one life form builds on another and just like embryology in which the development of one cell provides the context for the development of its neighbours and its successors.

(House of Lords, Official Record, 7 December 1989, col. 1020)

The image of one life-form building on another simultaneously depicts a progression and a displacement of one moment by the next. In building on another form, the new form is not seen simply to extend it, for the conditions of its reproduction are modified by what has already happened; rather it adds to and thus substitutes its own complexity for the form that preceded it.[4] The new form is both there and not there in its predecessor. But what kind of illumination is this?

A Mandelbrot set apparently emerges and re-emerges from the fractal realisation of the 'same' elements. So the collection of points that constitutes a Mandelbrot set remains a collection of points. What also remains are certain similarities. While every instantiation is produced out of the previous one, the same order of detail is kept throughout the scales. In that sense, the pattern at one stage is not more complex than at any other. Rather each magnification of detail replicates, though as the Archbishop observes in never quite the same way, detail visible at other orders of magnification. The same transformation is thus repeated at different scales. Yet the purpose of Habgood's analogy was to reveal the development of one state of being out of another, not what the repetition of a transformative rule could show.

The sequences of the mathematical set are, in truth, an odd analogy for complexification when the issue is that one starts off with one order of phenomena and ends up with another. But what about the way he uses it?

One may infer that the analogy with chaos theory was not intended to replicate one analogy by reference to another analogy nor to suggest that chaos theory and embryology were made out of the 'same' elements. They are not parallels in the real world. Rather, Habgood's was the (representational, foundational) strategy of supposing that *by his analogy he was illuminating something altogether different*. The facts of evolution and embryology have a real existence. In this view they are simply made to appear to the imagination in the analogy with the Mandelbrot set. When facts are made known through an exercise of the imagination, one might say they are modified ('developed') thereby. But two different orders of knowledge are involved. What becomes interesting about the Archbishop's analogy, then, is the manner in which the analogy was drawn. 'The phenomenality of meaning provides [the] apt parallel' (Wagner 1991: 166). In bringing the two semantic domains – chaos theory and embryology – together, the Archbishop provides a powerful *model* for the gradualists' mode of *interpretation* with respect to the relationship between early embryonic life and the fully developed human person.

The process of debate in which the parliamentarians were engaged acknowledged that language provided a description, no more nor less, in the same way as the legislative decisions would put the stamp of human resolve on what was and what was not to count as relevant. The parliamentarians were assisting themselves to understand a set of complex processes, and there was self-conscious reflection on the language they were using. The Archbishop's analogy brought the process of construction to everyone's attention. I have already surmised that he did not intend everything he said to be taken metaphorically and that it was a non-metaphoric order of phenomena he was illuminating by his metaphors. That presumption is endlessly repeated or replicated in the act of interpretation. The replication of possibilities for adding to knowledge in this way rests on an irreducibility between types of knowledge.

Now, at least as it has been explained to a lay audience (Gleick 1987), one way to determine whether or not points belong to a Mandelbrot set is through an operation that turns on an irreducible relationship, in this case between number and rule of operation.[5] However high the magnitude of calculation, the original figuration of complexity remains; a lay person might imagine it as a relationship between two orders of knowledge (number/rule).[6] While the operation is endlessly replicable, the results are not infinite; in graphic terms the patterns reapeat or fold back on themselves, as one might say the same cultural images recur at different points in argument.

Here I remain with the observation that the repetition or replication of an irreducible relationship between different orders of knowledge affords an interesting parallel to the repeated operations of the Mandelbrot set. But in producing new demonstrations of irreducibility, it is also possible to gloss over old ones. By way of emphasising the relationship of continuity between early embryonic life and human person in order to show that the latter is a developmental outcome of the former, the Archbishop produces discontinuity in *another* relationship, in this case between that process as a matter of empirical fact and the metaphor drawn from chaos theory. Empirical evidence and metaphoric illumination appear non-reducible to each other.

The metaphor is drawn upon by the Archbishop, reiterated by Morgan and Lee, in order to assist the understanding of complex issues at stake but not to suggest an intrinsic relationship between fractal geometry and reproduction. Insofar as the metaphor is not interrogated, it acquires a taken-for-granted facticity in the debate. However, this would not be a viewpoint shared by many indigenous Euro-Americans. They depict facticity through the ability to say something without having to have resort to metaphor, and a metaphor cannot (in this indigenous construction) therefore be a fact.

Types of parents

There is more than a formal correspondence between the Mandelbrot set and imagining the process of embryo development. For the anthropologist interested in the cultural facts that interpretation produces, there is also a substantive correspondence. That is, where it is grasped that embryo development is itself apprehended in the understanding or the representation of it, then grasping the mathematical analogy constitutes one mode of apprehension.

I am imagining that a certain indigenous model of interpretation is at stake. It consists in the view that the very act of understanding reproduces a difference between the naturally existing object of knowledge (facts to be stated) and the representational or artificial conventions of conceptual categories (interpretations to be made explicit). The difference could be called that between 'recognition' and 'construction'.[7] It is liable to appear whenever Euro-Americans think about what their knowledge represents. The distinction exists for example, at the heart of modernist Euro-American middle-class models of relations between certain kin. Between parent and child, the child is recognised; the parent, by contrast, is constructed.

By this I mean that the child is regarded as autonomously produced by biological processes in the same way as it is bound to grow into an autonomous adult (person). It does not even need to know its parents in order to exist as a child, though to be the child *of* someone depends on parentage. But that it has (had) parents is automatically presumed. To see a child is thus to 'recognise' a natural fact. Yet parents exist only through a double recognition: to recognise a parent is to have already recognised a child. For they exist only insofar as their children are *known* to exist, since persons are not presumed to be parents unless there is some way of knowing they have had children. Whether socially or legally, by contrast with the child, parenthood is thus always 'constructed' as an object of knowledge. As a consequence, the relationship *between* parent and child works as a hybrid, a kind of amalgam of different orders of fact.[8]

If we then look at the relationship between the parents, we encounter a similar hybrid. At least as far as mid-twentieth-century Euro-American kinship thinking is concerned, the category parent contains the same distinction within it. Betwen mother and father, the mother is recognised; the father, by contrast, is constructed.

I do not need to adduce examples of the extent to which Euro-Americans have regarded motherhood as a 'natural' phenomenon in a way that fatherhood must always be a 'social' or 'cultural' and in this sense artificial one [see Chapter 1]. It was long thought there was a certainty about the former (childbirth was the evidence) and a corresponding and intrinsic uncertainty about the latter (paternity could only ever be presumed). This was instantiated in law. 'In English law a husband is presumed to be the father of any child born to his wife unless it can be proved that he is not its natural father' (Wolfram 1987: 121). Indeed, the anthropology of kinship began in debates that arose from exactly this point. Whereas maternity was known through the obviousness of the birth process, paternity had to be inferred from the conjugal union. In short, the mother is constituted in her connection with the child, whereas the father is constituted in his relationship to the mother.

Each parent contributes their part to the process of procreation, but these are not parallel to each other. Any symmetry between them may also be subsumed under asymmetry. Thus while their genetic endowments are assumed to be similar, and are equally 'recognised' in their offspring, the inference was traditionally validated in different ways as far as the identity of a particular parent was concerned.[9]

In traditional Euro-American thinking, the mother's identity is created by her offspring in the act of her (visibly) giving birth. But the father is at a further remove. He is identified through the mother–child connection, that is, the mother's demonstrated connection to the child is prior to his claims with respect to the child. The certainty of the connection between mother and child is thus necessary to the certainty of the father's claim (cf. Cannell 1990: 673). Insofar as these claims turn on his relationship with the mother, they are regarded – in middle-class English kinship practice – as dependent on a social relationship. We should not be confused here by the issues of legality. The so-called 'natural' father has to demonstrate a 'social' relationship to the mother quite as much as the jural father whose paternity is established through marriage. In short, to see a mother is thus to recognise a natural connection, whereas conventionally speaking a man is not presumed to be a father unless there is some way of knowing about his connection with the mother. The identity of the father is thus constructed as a (conventional) object of knowledge.

But while this is true of the identiy of the parent, what about the substance of the tie itself? Can we agree further with Cannell (1990: 672, my emphasis) that 'biological mother *hood* and biological father *hood* are constructed in asymmetrical ways'? It is highly suggestive that new reproductive arrangements are able to make visible different possibilities that inhere in the *kind of relationship* seen to flow from the connection of substance.

Cannell is commenting on discussions about donor insemination as they appeared in the 1984 Warnock Report concerning the fact that fatherhood, by contrast with motherhood, is traditionally constituted in a genetic tie alone. The problem arises when *only* that tie is present. For different weight is put on the kind of relationship that flows from the combination of 'biological' facts. This means that the substance that makes a 'biological father' is not what makes a 'biological mother'. So while the biological (genetic) father is invariably referred to as a 'father' [Chapter 1], that person is not necessarily held to be a parent: there is uncertainty about what relationship the act of donation as such creates. Of course, one may argue that the same must hold for the donation of ova in isolation.

It is interesting to read therefore that, faced with this issue, members of the Warnock Committee offered different opinions about the desirability of semen and egg donation respectively, and regarded their implications for relationship differently (Haimes n.d.). This reiterates the asymmetry. When the comparison is between two types of donation, the very practice of genetic endowment may cease to seem similar.

Thus we have two types of parent and, potentially at least, two types of parenthood. Let me return to an older Euro-American formulation. 'Mothers are distinguished from fathers on the strength of biological correlates. Fathers represent culture whereas mothers represent nature' (Dolgin 1990: 526, references omitted). Now 'nature' and 'culture' are not divisions of a whole. Each term at once implies a separate domain and each also adds something to the other. Culture includes the cultural construction of natural facts; nature presents a facticity with which culture has to deal.[10] I see the same irreducibility in the Euro-American depiction of the difference between father and mother as between parent and child.

Between parent and child, one source of difference lies in the temporal direction of the relationship, insofar as the parent is thought to be prior (and the parent's genetic material to be the origin of the child's). Father and mother are not temporally separated by such a sequence. But they are separated by what one might call different temporalities of body process. The single act of the father is conventionally contrasted with the developmental involvement of the mother's physiology, from her initial receptivity to her bringing to term the growing foetus within her, and then to bodily and other forms of nurture once the baby is born.

In the same way as one might recognise different stages of embryo development, leading to the degree of complexity that constitutes the complete human being, so one might recognise different stages in the mother's involvement with the child. Each builds on the previous one: the mother in a complete sense is the hybrid outcome of complexification. She thus contains within her evidence of both 'natural' and 'cultural' facts. If gradualists think of the emergent foetus as recapitulating a movement from the recognition of natural fact (cellular formation) to the social construction of human meaning (person), so the mother, in this view, moves from what is ordinarily taken as a natural state (fertilisation) to a social one (the roles she takes on as nurturer). The latter state in turn recapitulates the dual process of recognition and construction. *In itself*, motherhood stands for the social construction of natural facts.

It is perhaps not surprising to find, therefore, that new parenting arrangements made possible by reproductive medicine suppose that different stages in maternal development have different meanings for motherhood. I refer particularly to the possibilities that IVF and other opportunities such as donor insemination afford what is known as maternal 'surrogacy'. Such possibilities in turn lead to new adjudication about what constitutes motherhood. Frequently represented as a splitting apart of maternal functions that were formerly combined in the one person, the fragmenting of the figure of the mother can also, I suggest, be interpreted processually. Decisions turn not on the stage of complexity that development has reached, as in the case of the embryo; rather, they present the inverse case, how one can divide up an already complex entity in order to determine which component has the most weight. This is the undoing, we might say, of a developmental model.

Here it is the continuities that are glossed over in the necessity to distinguish the different parts that make up the figure of the mother. Once set in motion there seems no end to the process of partition. The effect is (in this case) not development but division.

Division cannot be symmetrical. We may expect it to replicate the asymmetrical adding of different orders of knowledge to each other. Indeed, we find that different weights are put on different components of the maternal role, most broadly distinguished as social and biological. An asymmetrical relationship, then, is not to be simply prised apart. Partition makes apparent the discontinuity between social construction and natural fact. Each recovers its own irreducibility.

Mandelbrot in Melanesia

There is nothing in Melanesian formulations to suggest that Melanesians think of kinship as the social construction of natural facts. We might ask, therefore, what Mandelbrot is doing there. For one recent understanding of kinship has discovered Mandelbrot in Melanesia. As the previous chapter indicates, Wagner (1991) draws on fractal geometry as a way of restating how people there visualise reproduction. Where, then, is irreducibility?

In the Melanesian case, such motivation is not to be found in the difference between mother and father, or child and parent, by which Euro-Americans confront themselves with different orders of knowledge (fact and interpretation, recognition and construction). On the contrary, mother and father, like child and parent, are reducible: each can appear as a version of the other. The irreducible entity is not the type of parent or type of person; it is the person and his/her relationships.

A person's relations are at once integral to him/her and carried by him/her. They form an irreducible entity insofar as that integral relationship is repeated whenever Melanesians encounter either persons or relations – the one is not replicated without the other. A 'fractal person' is thus a person with a relationship implied. As a consequence, a person in a relationship (as Euro-Americans would express it), e.g. a mother or father, is analogous to any other person in a relationship. As concepts, each can work as a metaphor for the other.

Kinship becomes a flow of analogies.[11] Thus Wagner characterises a range of non-Euro-American kinship systems (his type case is from Papua New Guinea) as being founded on an analogical approach:

> Having obviated the distinction between 'natural' kin type and 'cultural' kin relationship by subsuming terminology and relationship within a single entity, an analogical approach does not incorporate the contrast between 'mental' symbolization and 'physical' fact. Its constructions are intended as simultaneously conceptual and phenomenal; they belong to a single universe of apprehended cultural construction (and culturally constructed apprehension) that is contiguous with other realms of conceptualization.
>
> (Wagner 1977: 626–7)

Now in that Melanesians take analogy for granted, it does not and cannot have the constructionist force it carries in systems that rest on a difference between recognition and construction.

What the figure of a fractal person contains are other persons: he or she is a person with other persons implied in his/her constitution [cf. Chapter 4]. Reproduction in this regime turns out to be an act of differentiation, one that divides persons from persons in such a way as to create differences between domains or dimensions. We could say that in an analogic system irreducibility is not assumed but must be created by convention.

In approaching them through a relationship between different orders of knowledge, modern Euro-Americans find mother and father to be irreducibly different. Each parent appears to belong to a different domain or dimension (prototypically, nature/culture). What is thus re-created each time is exactly this knowledge: the difference is discovered afresh in the particulate identity of each figure. It is modernist knowledge practices themselves that afford analogies for the way differentiations are endlessly repeated, as I have tried to indicate, and are re-created every time one tries to 'know' something. For the difference between orders of knowing (recognition, construction) is a relation integral to such knowledge. We might even say that the same order of complexity is repeated in each instance of this relationship. That is why I have insisted that the appropriate analogy for the Mandelbrot set lies, for Euro-Americans, in the act of interpretation itself. It is the misfortune of interpretation, like culture [Chapter 3], to appear as artificial as analogies and metaphors always do in this system.

But here in Melanesia people seemingly take the analogical process for granted and see it manifest in the recursive repetition of persons. In other words, persons inevitably stand in a metaphoric relationship to other persons. Irreducibility *between* persons/relations is a momentary outcome of differentiation. That being so, social life consists in creating differentiations (dividing person from person, relations from relations), and Melanesians accomplish this in their constant partitioning of themselves [Chapter 5]. It is the act that differentiates. Thus actions are constantly being framed off from one another to 'transformative'[12] effect − as in the events anthropologists identify as childbirth, bridewealth, ceremonial exchange, war compensation, sister-exchange, male initiation, female seclusion, and the rest.

When a person is conceived fractally, then, relationships are already implied; one parent is already a version or metaphor of, and in his or her relations analogous to, another parent, and the work of convention is that of differentiation. What have to be established are particularities of identity, those individual facts that Euro-American constructions take for granted. Differentiation consists in making distinctions between different types or versions of the 'same' thing. Establishing origins, for instance, is a Melanesian way of establishing a distinction between types of parent or types of children. One parent may be seen as originating from ancestral parents whereas the second parent's ancestry may cease to be carried forward. That in turn will be repeated in the differentiation of children, between those who do and who do not replicate the parent. Fatherhood and motherhood remain metaphors for each other, in this thinking, in the same way as either continuity or discontinuity with the past constitute analogous reference points (origins), or brothers' sons are analogous to sisters' sons. Differentiations have to be imagined as significant moments or events (acts) that sever one type of relationship from another.

Thus we have two types of parent, but as divisions of one type of parenthood. Different orders of knowledge ('nature' and 'culture') are not involved; rather a partitioning of what can be apprehended as a single person/relation into analogous – similar but not identical – versions of itself. How might this be imagined?

It can be imagined in the division and duplication of body substance at conception. The Baruya of interior Papua New Guinea, for example, suppose that there is really only 'one' substance that produces persons, semen, but that it is divided into different forms (Godelier 1986: 52). Thus mothers are different from and at the same time versions of fathers by virtue of the fact that they pass on semen in the female form of milk. They are metaphoric fathers! The difference is that whereas mother's milk nourishes, father's semen both builds the body and has a potency that can itself also be passed on. Mother's ancestry is not carried forward in the way that father's is. While semen is thus divided into male and female versions, it can also be replenished and duplicated when, in becoming adults, boys and girls alike are given fresh doses of semen in addition to that which they received from their parents.[13]

This difference between parents is remade when boys are partitioned from girls through initiation rituals; the rituals ensure that what differentiates boys from girls is the way in which they process semen. Once separated from girls, boys then find they are partitioned internally: their bodies, it is revealed, are made up of two kinds of semen – that which forms their bodily tissue (bones, flesh) and that which they contain within themselves to transmit to their own offspring. They are thus doubly constituted of the same substance.[14] What the father-to-be passes on is a transmissible version of the substance that constitutes his own body but is not transmissible. The male child thus replicates within himself the same division that divides mother from father. He is composed of substance that stays with him (as the mother nourishes her child) and of substance that can be passed on (as the father does).

We might say that for the Baruya semen itself contains that relationship within it (divided between the transmissible and non-transmissible parts). It is fractually realised, both within the person (made up of different kinds of semen) and between persons (who have different kinds of parents made from semen).

Baruya operations thereby create two types of parent, even though the actions of each have the same effect on the child which is ultimately to turn him or her into a parent himself or herself. Persons are either divided from one another or duplicated, as the vitalising substance Baruya men circulate among themselves is divided and duplicated. The difference between the two types of parent is established through people's actions. For parents-to-be − of either sex − evince that difference in their bodies: the strength given them by paternal semen transformed by their mothers into nourishing milk, and that given them directly by other men so they can reproduce. Division and duplication is contained within. The same order of complexity is therefore replicated in every appearance and realisation of 'semen', whether of one person, of a couple, or of the whole Baruya tribe (cf. Godelier n.d.). Complexity does not 'increase' as in the processual Euro-American model of embryo development.

Indeed, there is no theory of development here; rather, each type of substance implies the other. Transmissible and non-transmissible forms of semen between them reproduce the person in a relationship. Both sexes are the completed outcome of the acts of others.

Baruya men make this very apparent to themselves in their insistence that to render boys into potent fathers they must add semen to semen; but what is added is simultaneously divided. It is thought there is a finite stock of the substance partible between the men. It can be replenished − even as men's bodies are nurtured by milk − but when Baruya men look at a multitude of boys they are also looking at fractional realisations of the one substance. Each boy in turn, as we have seen, contains that fractioning within himself. A man is thus both 'mother' and 'father', so to speak, until he acts as 'father' to a woman who will 'mother' his child. The boy becomes a father when he partitions himself in the act of intercourse through which transmissible semen is released to form a new person. Persons and relations, like bodies, are partible.

Through similar imaginative devices, a Baruya women is partitioned at childbirth. In fact, the very act of childbirth is regarded as divisive: the semen the mother received from her father is retained in her own body while the semen she received from her husband becomes the body of the child. Releasing the child divides one person from another person (father from husband), one relation from another relation, and thus one kind of father (her own father) from another kind of father (her child's father).

The partition of the parent

In the way in which the splitting apart of maternal functions are represented in Euro-American talk about surrogacy, however, the language is not of division and duplication but of fragmentation – and that is because the maternal body was never partible. It was constituted in what it combined, not in how it could be divided. In this sense, it was always a composite: the social construction of natural facts.[15] Different functions of the maternal body could be compared to different stages of embryonic development, as I have done; yet, as analogies, the parallels between fertilisation and parturition or between the functions of the natural body and the social construction of motherhood must remain partial. These were, above all, stages in a process, the combining of elements that cohered as a complex matter of development.

The distinctiveness of the embryo is a component of this worldview, a unique composite body contained wihin the mother's that will in its own development duplicate the relationship between nature and culture. Like the Baruya child, then, the Euro-American child reproduces within himself or herself two types of parent – the one that represents 'nature' and the one that represents 'culture'. Yet these are not partible components of the 'same' thing. Rather, they are grafted on to each other in the view of developmental sequence and biological/cultural process in such a way that the completed child is the cultural or social construction of a natural fact.

In Euro-American convention a body taken apart is neither divided nor duplicated: it is more likely to be thought of as mutilated. Part from whole does not so much create two entities out of one as dismember the original; partition is inevitably unequal. Different orders of being are derived from parts and wholes, even as different orders of knowledge are added in the recognition and construction of facts.

To return to an earlier observation, gamete donation does not divide parental functions between persons. But it can be seen as adding and subtracting 'cells' from/to 'persons'. It is precisely because cells and persons remain incommensurable that questions are raised about what parenthood should be. Cells are literally body parts.

The imagery of fragmentation is pervasive. Braidotti regards contemporary bioscience as taking the body as a mosaic of detachable pieces (1988: 152): organs without bodies. Fragmentation, in her view, is everywhere. The reproductive process is broken into a series of discontinuous steps, parenting into different degrees of nurturance. 'Swapping the totality for the parts that compose it, ignoring the fact that each part contains the whole, the era of "bodies without organs" is primarily the era that has pushed time out of the bodily picture' (1988: 153). She sees the 'ever-receding fragmentation and traffic in organ parts' as denying time in the denial of generational difference: 'my uterus, my mother's uterus' (1988: 157). Indeed, in her view, it thereby encourages *false* symmetries, both between the generations and between men and women.[16] The idea of fragmentation evokes a counterpart idea of some prior whole. Yet if conceptually speaking the whole was always a composite, a hybrid, it could never disperse into anything but unequal fragments. Symmetries become false indeed.

There is no symmetry between the different types of mothers created through surrogacy arrangements. As Dolgin states (1990: 526, emphasis omitted), 'mothers can be opposed to other kinds of mothers'. Some come to represent culture, some nature (the commissioning or contract mother as opposed to the genetic and/or birth mother).

Dolgin addresses the legal issues in the Baby M case brought before the New Jersey courts in 1988. Although the legal dispute lay between the genetic and commissioning father and the surrogate mother, its interest in the present context lies in her exposition of the differences between the mothers' claims. As between the two 'mothers' (the commissioning mother, and the surrogate who was also the genetic mother) the two claims to motherhood were irreducible. The former was based in law; the latter in biology. It was not, of course, quite as simple as that: thus the commissioning mother also had a natural claim based on the desirability of reproducing traditional family life, a social one based on her marriage to the father, and so on. But while Dolgin's concern is to show how 'mixed' the law becomes in applying criteria from both domains, we have seen that irreducible difference already there in the figure of the mother who evinces both nature and culture in her very constitution. There is no symmetry between the identities of genetic, birthing, or commissioning mother.[17] Body parts split, the maternal figure is fragmented: the violent language of some commentators is appropriate because Euro-American persons were never partible. What have to be prised apart in surrogacy arrangements are components of what was originally thought of as combining in a single continuous process of mothering.

Present-day possibilities allow a mode of interpretation that brings Baruya practice to mind. One can nowadays be seen to *act* on the differentiation of the maternal figure into her natural and social/cultural attributes; indeed one can apparently 'duplicate' motherhood by locating each in a different person. Yet there is no duplication of rights and claims. What have to be partitioned are not divisions of a single substance or identity or person − but a complex being developed from components none of which is reducible to, or a simple version of, the others. So an asymmetry remains. Euro-Americans are uncertain as to how to 'divide' motherhood. The difficulties that arose in the Bay M case testify both to the irreducibility of the elements involved and to the way in which till now they have been held to modify or supplement one another.

* * *

Mandelbrot's set does, indeed, illuminate the way Euro-Americans' interpretations constantly combine and recombine with whatever facts are under debate. Were one to think of Modell's intervention [Chapter 7], however, one might think of another metaphor for the coming into being of human life. It would suppose an analogy between two kinds of persons.

The complexity involved in embryonic formation, when each stage is seen as the point from which a different stage develops, as in the end the person is regarded as different from but also the outcome of the original cellular form, is not to be apprehended through the simple imagery of growth precisely because at every point it manifests a different set of potentials for its natural and social (cultural) future. And these two are never of equal weight; they are always asymmetrical. It was that asymmetrical combination of identities that made the embryology debate complex. This is not unlike the way that Euro-American kinship has in the past imagined the person of the mother.

The mother's role unfolds with the formation, birth and care of the child, and in attending to its needs perceived as both natural and social she is herself defined by the asymmetrical combination of natural and social functions. Yet 'motherhood' comes into being not potentially but actually at the moment of conception.[18] In that sense, the traditional figure of the mother is after all a poor analogy for the continuously emergent aspects of developmental process, the gradualism Habgood was also talking about. But what is newly available for us to think with is her potential partition.[19] Surrogacy arrangements decombine elements, substitute discontinuity for continuity, un-do the hybrid, reverse process. Devolution rather than development: the new figure of the dispersible mother. The figure is made new by the way we think it. In seeing how we are able to take that once complex person apart, we might better understand the imaginative procedures by which we put together its embryonic precursor.

Notes

1 I am grateful to Sarah Franklin for bringing his distinction to my attention; she did so in the context of her own study of the parliamentary debates, and her insights have contributed to the present chapter.

2 Other speakers had argued that the conditions for uniqueness were laid down with the unique union of genetic material at 'fertilisation'.

3 Chapter 1 argued that discussion over human beginnings can, when it is taken as a matter of biological development, proceed without reference to social factors, by contrast with legal debate over who shall be regarded as the social parents, which must proceed with some reference to natural factors. Here what is at issue are those human beginnings themselves, and the same asymmetry is repeated on a different scale. For those who promote the gradualist view, cellular development can be recognised without reference to social factors, but the debate over the social significance of the degree of complexity must proceed with reference to the natural ones. One should, however, note, and the point recurs in Chapter 8, that the social language of individuality already gives a prospective cast to the biological language of cellular identity.

4 Chaos theory, which claims Mandelbrot's set as one of its exemplars, involves the non-linear modelling of the regular but essentially unpredictable emergence of phenomena. We could say the Archbishop was

conveying a non-linear model of complexity, when his audience might have in their minds a model of embryo growth as a matter of simple linear progression. Best (1991) offers an excellent analysis of the relationship of chaos theory to other exemplifications of postmodern thought.

5 The initial number is apparently a two-dimensional complex number, that is, already composed of elements in different planes as one might imagine a point on a grid reference mapped by two directions. (I add that I should disclaim any mathematical knowledge on my part in the manner that many of the parliamentary speakers disclaimed knowledge of embryology or science.)

6 What is of interest for the present argument about the way we present knowledge to ourselves is that each change of scale – the magnitude of phenomena under scrutiny – reintroduces both the same complexity and the same substantive asymmetries. The point can be illustrated through a familiar paradox. If you imagine someone at the midpoint along a path, and then imagine him or her at the midpoint along the next half of that, and at the midpoint again along the next half, the traveller would never reach his or her destination. The paradox is that we know that, of course, he/she will, even though he/she passes each midpoint exactly as described. The solution is to see that the *imagining* of this process involves a fractal extension. That is, at each juncture, two different orders or dimensions are being brought together, and it is that conjunction that is repeated over and again in the posing of the paradox. When we are invited to imagine something half-way along its path, and then half-way along what is left, we are not proceeding along a straight line at all: the first half is not the same as the second half. The first half is half the whole length; the second half is half of a different length altogether, that is, the length that was left. Two different lengths are thus being combined (a divided and an undivided length). At each juncture a 'new' one is added to an 'old' one. What is irreducible – and what means that this *line of thinking* will never get the traveller to his/her destination – is the imagined replication of that relationship between old and new lengths.

7 I adopt the late modernist term 'construction' as ethnographically appropriate for the middle-class Euro-American (positivist) discourse I have been elucidating in these essays. By *recognition* I mean that the activity of the imagination is regarded as being exercised in order to bring to the imagination facts that are not regarded as dependent upon it. Thus Mandelbrot's set is brought to bear on the natural facts of embryo growth as a way of forcing people to a certain realisation. We might say that what is recognised is always already there in the language of factuality and information; the process of recognition simply involves the imaginative accessing of information. In *construction*, however, this world-view holds that human decisions have to intervene in the description of events

in order to create categories that can then be acted upon. Thus the care with which the concept of person was, for many speakers in the parliamentary debate, reserved for a late stage of human growth reflected a self-consciousness about the jural implications of using such a term. Such a construction, it was openly recognised, was a social convention. The perception of the natural facts (recognition) can act as a ground or reference point for decisions about what social conventions (constructions) should apply. At the same time, conventions can be seen as transformations of facts — facts being put to human use — and thus as continuous with and as having their 'origin' in facts. As with fact and interpretation, then, recognition and construction (precept and concept; perceptual image and referential code; 'number' and 'rule') are, depending on context, mutually encompassing terms. Either 'construction' or 'recognition' may serve as the higher-order term which encompasses the distinction between them. However, I do not pursue these issues here.

8 A child is, we might say, 'added' to a couple in making them parents, even as partners are 'added' to each other to form a parental pair.

9 I am grateful to David Schneider for reminding me of the difference between what a parent is and who a parent is: he argues (pers. comm.) that genetic endowment and the act of sexual intercourse define motherhood and fatherhood symmetrically. However, he allows that knowing who the mother and who the father is may rest on an asymmetry in how that knowledge is acquired. I take the latter point rather further in the argument that follows.

10 Culler (1979: 168) notes that Rousseau's delineation of this particular relationship was a source for the Derridean concept of supplementation.

11 'Consider, then, a situation in which all kin relations and all kinds of relatives are basically alike, and it is a human responsibility to differentiate them. The responsibility of doing so will be our task in understanding kin relationships, as it is man's role in perhaps the majority of human societies. A mother is another kind of a father, fathering is another kind of mothering' (Wagner 1977: 623).

12 Transformation is not apprehended as development [but see further the next chapter]. One does not add different domains of activity to each other but converts one into the other (e.g. political into domestic action). The account here is much simplified. 'Differentiation', for instance, covers two processes, distinguishable as (same-sex) duplication/division and (cross-sex) production of one form out of another (transformation). That gender difference is a source of Melanesian asymmetry (Strathern 1988).

13 As Godelier (1986) describes, boys are inseminated by their elders; girls are fed with milk by women, then with semen by their new husbands. It is of interest to add that cultural neighbours of the Baruya, Ankave, similarly conceptualise the duplication and division of substance, but in

this case the substance is blood not semen (Bonnemère n.d.). Blood takes various forms, though it appears neither as milk (its nourishing counterpart) nor as semen. The mother converts food into blood, and her blood into food for the baby as well as filling the foetus up with its own blood. 'Blood', in the form of red pandanus juice, is applied to boy initiates to make them grow. Ties of substance and nurture are conceptualised as blood ties, and flow from the mother; though Ankave are, like Baruya, 'patrilineal' in group organisation, in the Ankave case continuity of substance is determined through women. Bonnemère comments that clan organisation is thus discontinuous from relations based on body substance. The contrast between Baruya and Ankave invites comparison with that of Beti and Samo discussed by Houseman (1988). I am most grateful to Maurice Godelier and to Pascale Bonnemère for allowing me to cite from unpublished papers.

14 Each boy also has 'two' fathers: the sun and his human father (Godelier 1986: 51). It might seem as though I am overlooking the contribution that the mother's 'flesh' is said to make to the formation of the foetus, but that flesh is itself transformed (paternal) semen.

15 Like 'kinship' itself [again, refer back to Chapter 1]. In this sense motherhood is homologous to kinship.

16 I also draw on Braidotti's observations in another context, in a contribution to a seminar convened by Lawrence Rosen on *The Cultural Analysis of Intentionality* (Sante Fe, 1990).

17 Where the commissioning mother is also the genetic mother, she may be described as the 'biological' as opposed to the 'host' (carrying) mother (*Daily Telegraph* 6.8.91).

18 That is, with respect to her relationship to the embryo-to-be there is no other way to think of her but as a mother, exactly because a *relationship* is at issue and because she is already a person. (Mothers may be called incubators, and all sorts of other things, but such imaery has nothing to do with the stage of embryonic or foetal development.) It may not be complete motherhood that she enacts, but it has no other identity.

19 The dovetailing of development with both change and continuity is another, though far from new, possibility, and is explored in the next chapter.

CHAPTER 8

Reproducing anthropology

Thought of the future is momentous; but why wish to project forward? Since we know one can only extrapolate from present concerns, what does it mean to ask where anthropology is going? Is it in order to imagine ways in which present concerns might also be part of the future's past, the beginnings of something still to grow, an origin point for posterity?

What is certainly momentous about the future is that it will determine its own genealogy — will ignore Haddon and revere Rivers, or forget Hutton and respect Fortes. It is in such expectation that we perhaps wish to bring forward some intimation of what *will be* significant. Anticipating how paradigms tumble and intellectual fashions pass makes investment in the present uncertain, and prompts curiosity about what will emerge. Once one knew, one could act! One would be in a position to discount surface babble and detect new voices. Otherwise there is the terrible thought that we might be going down the wrong road or putting eggs into the wrong basket; that endeavours might lead nowhere and ideas bear no fruit. Suppose there is no flowering of the discipline? The future would have killed us off.

Origins and links

Evolutionary narrative tells of obscure beginnings; chaos theory suggests how the faintest perturbations in the air may affect continental weather patterns, and newspaper-reading Westerners are constantly invited to reflect on the making of global events out of local ones. Journalists sometimes anticipate the reflection, and then news comes as already history. Indeed, there is a sense in which significance inevitably lies in what things become, for it is only the retrospective light that picks them out at all.

Such was the future that Ortner, for example, saw in those

past developments in anthropology that had led to then current theoretical preoccupations. She wrote: 'in order to understand the significance of this trend ... we must go back at least twenty years and see where we started from, and how we got to where we are now' (1984: 127). The journeying metaphor suggests that to know where to start from depends not only on pinpointing a significant origin − it also depends on sustaining a *link* between that point and those who value it. When the origins of ideas are attributed to individual persons, the link may be imagined as the transmission of knowledge. It 'develops' thereby. Fortes (1969) thus constructed a line of succession between himself, Radcliffe-Brown, Rivers and Morgan. Ideas, formulations, analytical practices are, in this view, passed on from teacher to pupil or author to reader, transmitted from mind to mind as an unfolding sequence of links from some original practice or statement. So if genealogies are traced up, then knowledge is seen as flowing down − whether handed on by the possessor of it or inherited inadvertently by one who only later uncovers the origins of his or her own reflections.

These observations seem commonplace. Causes have effects and acts have consequences, to which can be added other unremarkable facts such that development is irreversible, transmission links donor and recipient and life moves from the simple to the complex. Commonplaces are grounded in taken-for-granted knowledge about the world.

It is not knowledge, however, that everyone takes for granted. The discourse which supposes that ideas may be traced to their origins in individual persons, for instance, enlists the authentication of 'presence' that Derridean-inspired criticism has long regarded as endorsing a very particular metaphysics. The question becomes how discourses achieve their effects. Here I merely observe that practices of authentication are bound to recur in diverse cultural loci. Identifying a locus is, of course, like finding an origin. One makes it significant. The cultural locus I have in mind (wish to make significant) embeds the ideas of origins in the idea of developmental process. As we shall see, it already queries the kinds of decisions that can be made about what is 'present' at any one time; the processual nature of development, however, is simply taken as a fact.

The locus I call a 'reproductive model' (after Yeatman 1983); a model of procreative process, it is also a model for the future.

It is found in discourse characteristically middle-class (mid-)twentieth-century and Euro-American.

The model consists in certain representations of the relation between development and heredity. The terms I borrow from the embryologist, Grobstein, speaking at a recent debate intended among other things to broaden public understanding of scientific matters. Either term may encompass the difference between them; thus he divides 'heredity' into two constitutive components. Hereditary material (DNA) has an effect either when it is replicated (as a genotype or genome) or when the genotype is in turn expressed (as a phenotype).[1] 'The first process is the foundation of heredity, the second is correspondingly the foundation of development. Together the two constitute reproduction in all living organisms' (Grobstein 1990: 15). He went on to remark: 'As understanding of heredity has emerged, first through accumulated experience and then through increasingly sophisticated science, it has been integrated into various technological practices ... It has also taken root in our dominant attitudes and habits of thought' (1990: 16). I suggest that the process of taking root includes the way in which such understanding is 'replicated' and 'expressed' in understandings of social relationships between persons. These include the domain of kinship as it is construed by many Euro-Americans. Such 'kinship' is not independent of the facts of reproduction as the embryologist presents them, but it also draws on other areas of experience and knowledge, as well as being drawn upon as a resource for thinking about other relationships. If we consider these domains as different loci of authentication, then one relation between them is that of analogy.

The reproductive model plays off heredity and development through a contrast between the relationships implied in parenting and ancestry and the individuality that must be claimed by and for the child as the outcome of these relationships.[2]

Consider a feature that Macfarlane (e.g. 1986: 82) has identified as characteristic of English kin-reckoning. This is the downward flowing or descending nature of obligations and emotions which means that a parent has greater future concern for the child than a child has a backward duty to the parent (and cf. Finch 1989: 53). The child's physical origins lie in the bodies of others, a link as indissoluble as its own genetic formation is normally deemed irreversible. Yet parents only reproduce parts of themselves. Like the fortune one may or may not be born into, the conjunction of genetic traits is assumed to be fortuitous. While the child claims its origins in its parents' make-up, it itself evinces a unique combination of characteristics, and the combination is regarded as a matter of chance. This lays the basis of its individuality. Individuality is thus a significant outcome of relationships – indeed parents are expected to assist the child to develop that independence which is one manifestation of it (hence the lesser expectation of duty). At the same time, 'individuals' must also be seen as making themselves. Although the basis for the link between parent and child lies in the child's past, what that link will mean in the future is contingent on how the individual person acts. The nature of interaction, the degree of obligation felt, and in respect of lateral connections through the parent even whether a tie is acted on at all (cf. Firth and Djamour 1956; Firth *et al.* 1969), all depend on what the child will *make* of its past.

Such Euro-American kinship constructs thus evoke ideas about change and continuity, either of which can apply to the development of organisms or to hereditary transmission.

As an aspect of development, continuity is imaginable as a ceaseless process or extension, in the same way as a child grows imperceptibly from one stage to the next. Change, by contrast, comes from the way development acts upon or from within an organism[3] such that what was one thing becomes, and perhaps quite radically, another with its own distinctive characteristics. Thus it is half expected that branches of a family will grow apart in terms of fortune and social status. Discontinuities will be understood as the effect of accumulated small changes; knowing what point of a road one is upon establishes distinctive identity. As an aspect of heredity, on the other hand, change appears evident in every new generation, unique with respect to its forebears in evincing a radical combination of earlier characteristics. Continuity is imaginable as genetic inheritance, the transmission of markers of identity that create links between the present generation and past ones. Talents are traceable to this or that person or branch of the family, though only some points of origin are recalled and others are dropped from history. Continuity expresses a link of identity, and to discover an origin for some aspect of one's identity replicates the link itself.

These perceptions are problematised in a multitude of fields, from periodisation in history and speciation in zoology to adjudication on social and cultural boundaries.[4] But perhaps it is a model such as this which prompts the projections of academics and anthropologists: the hope that original ideas will make a radical impression on the future — provided, that is, some kind of continuous link can be maintained with the present that will be its past!

Discontinuities

One characteristic of the relation between heredity and development is that each element is held to activate the other. As concepts, each also encompasses the difference between them, as is true of the pairs of ideas I have extrapolated from the reproductive model. For the difference between continuity and change repeats itself in terms of differences within each. An intriguing example is Gellner's (1964) differentiation of evolutionary and episodic time as modalities of change. The reference comes from McDowell's (1985) development of his concept of episodic time with respect to Melanesian ethno-history. An episodic view imagines sudden, catastrophic transformations as opposed to continual, developmental ones. Now the episodic view, which she suggests characterises much Melanesian thinking about change, is not confined to distinctions between mythic pasts and timeless presents; transformations are also attributed to social discontinuities between persons.

We could expect a comparison with the Euro-American reproductive model insofar as Melanesians calibrate their episodic view with formulations of growth and increment.[5] But they construct developmental process and thus the significance of past and future to rather different effect. If it is the Euro-American investment in origins and links that renders past and future of momentous significance to each other, the Melanesian view is (obviously) 'other' to this statement.

Peoples of the Papua New Guinea Highlands have their own models of procreation. Where in these patrilineal systems flutes constitute the revelatory heart of male initiation, they activate a flow of procreative power between men. Yet men's power is celebrated in the fact that initially the flutes were *not* theirs.[6] In mythic times, flutes existed only as the appendages of women; they came into men's hands through women's carelessness and men's cunning, at once a catastrophic break with the former epoch, and a transformation of identity — from thenceforth men possessed powers of procreation. But simple possession has not made these powers available for transmission to junior generations. Initiands must afresh face the hazard that when it is their turn they may fail to detach themselves properly from 'women', and fail to realise the potential of their masculinity.

In sum, possession is no guarantee of the ability to transmit; identity implies a radical break with the past; and a child must be detached from part of its ancestry. The origin of male potency thus lies in those who are not men, in persons now without the power they once had. A cultural corollary is that simply to be an origin does not make one significant in any other respect than that.[7] The past is not carried forward.

This is a special instance of a general state of affairs in men's relations with women. The hazard that every new generation of males encounters in having to detach themselves speaks of women's primordial power; however once detachment is effected, women's powers become trivial. The reproduction of exogamous patrilineal clans supplements this fact. Since a clan realises its fertility in the persons of wives whose origins are elsewhere, its significant powers are those of inducement, including the (bride)wealth it will transmit to these other (bride-giving) clans. The significance is claimed by men setting themselves off from women. Such transmission does not, however, create a link of continuity. Rather, to be a donor or recipient with respect to another separates the parties by their relationship [see Chapter 6].

When a woman is detached from her paternal clan, an internal displacement of identity ensures that her body will yield the child not of her father's clan but of her husband's. She is doubly the vehicle without which male procreative power could not be realised. This is also a special instance of a more general state of affairs: that forms appear out of 'other' forms. Whatever identity is claimed through lineal ancestors, coming into being also requires an originator with whom one does not share that identity – the stranger parent, the processing body.

Denial of 'identity' may be explicit. Persons can spend their lives paying for* their origins, confirming that the link they have with other kin consists in the discontinuity between them. When

---

* An example of the point made in the Introduction concerning an association between kinship sentiment and the making of payments.

non-lineal kin receive bridewealth and funeral payments, their claims on the outcome of their own procreative potency are thereby turned back, even killed one might say. That potency is being realised in 'other' persons. In some matrilineal regimes, a child carries an imprint of its father (and see A. Weiner 1983); but the matrilineal identity that appears in the form of the children of men must in the end be reclaimed by its originators. It is thus possible to reverse the flow of potency, and for a person to be divested of relationships that once composed him or her. And for there to be a future, the very dead may have to be 'killed' (e.g. Clay 1986: 121).[8] The living detach themselves from the (future) effects of the deceased who will no longer, in this sense, be the origin of their own acting.

If this is indeed a Melanesian model for the future, it imagines causes that cease to take effect, developments that can be put into reverse, a kinship that can be decomposed [and see Chapter 5]. Insofar as the social relationships that composed a deceased person must now be carried by others, in some Melanesian societies people actually undo links made in previous generations in order that future generations may forge new links. Each death is treated as the end of a social epoch. Land claims, house sites, personal names, whatever passage of time is required for their social transformation, the person is catastrophically dismantled.

Mortuary feasts organised by the Tanga of New Ireland (Foster 1990) make the point. The kin of the deceased both commemorate and 'finish' the person by reversing the direction of the links that nurtured him or her. A Tanga child grows up through being fed from the products of its father's matrilineage: at death members of this lineage are made to eat of the products of the deceased's own matrilineage, in return for which they give durable valuables.[9] The final act of the nurturant paternal lineage, then, is to create the durability and singularity of the deceased's lineage through agreeing to be the consumer in the relationship; the donor of the food is made impervious. Foster emphasises (and see Battaglia 1990: 195) the mutual dependence of matrilineages on one another for their enduring definitions as (after Dumont) collective individuals.

The feasts are also said to 'replace' the deceased (Foster 1990: 435). A maternal nephew parades with valuables given in the name of a deceased man to signify the future of the lineage. But the future is indeed the collective individual – the matrilineage shorn of exogenous relationships. Shorn thus, such individuals have no supports, no sources of nurture, no origins outside themselves. If life is only created in the supports, then they (individuated lineages) are not in that sense 'alive'. Indeed, no living person is an individual. To be alive as a person means to be the outcome of the acts of others, including others with whom no enduring identity is shared. A person cannot develop out of himself or herself in this model. Rather, persons exist to the extent that they activate their supports as a differentiated field of social relationships.

If living persons are produced out of the bodies (nurturance) of others than themselves, the same is true generally in Melanesia of people's plans and projects, including their intentions for the future. One's ideas are regarded not so much as transmitted as coming to fruition in the minds and acts of other persons. The effect that a person has constitutes the realisation of intention. Yet that realisation is by convention processed through another's gesture, another's pain. All outcomes are chancy in that an agent never knows quite what the effect of an action will be, and all are subject to being embodied in 'other' persons who make the effect appear. As a consequence, one seeks to make an impression on those who register the significance of what one does.

The future is known by what will endure of the identity of persons. At the same time, discontinuities between social persons also constitute potential discontinuities between present and future (or past) effects. Hence it is possible to bring the future into the present through social action. This is done every time a donor becomes a recipient or kin are paid off, as it is through those innovative decisions to kill all the pigs or change the marriage rules that will make a 'new time' come up (cf. McDowell 1985: 34). The future may thus be reordered by a radical rearrangement of relationships, as evinced in cargo cults and micronationalist movements (May 1982). The very possibility underwrites a substantive difference between it and the present. The present appears the more problematic. For since the effects of one's acts are always, contingently, in the hands of others, unlike the future the present is not open to reordering.

What the future will tell is how to evaluate the present. So it is the present rather than the future which is the momentous unknown. Only after the event can it be seen what kind of support one has. Once one has acted, one will know! What is already known about the future is what will endure, and that makes it, like the past, 'dead', without the supports of the living. For what endures, in this Melanesian view, will be already existing collective individuals such as clans and lineages – provided, that is, their identity is shorn of the vital effects of the present.

Anticipation

Among the Euro-American modes in which to think about the development of disciplines, I have suggested we might consider a reproductive model of origins and links. In its scholarly version it endorses a necessary relation between change (individual and unique works) and continuity (the transmission of concepts and theories). The possibility that one might have arrived at a crucial point in the unfolding of events, combined with the idea that the past will inform the future, leads to the conclusion that *anticipation is also potentiation*: once we know where we are, we can act.

Uncertainty about the present does not contrast with the future, in this view, so much as derive from it. It is how she sees 1980s anthropology 'taking shape' (1984: 158) that gives Ortner the current question to which her overview leads,[10] and one might be tempted to compare this with the anticipatory way Melanesians seek to draw the future into the present. But the parallel is not exact: the Euro-American view rests on the desirability of sustaining links.[11] If one overthrows an immediate intellectual ancestor, one is likely to reinstate an antecedent; the urgency is to identify the right origins with which to make the link. But insofar as choice in the matter is also desirable, one does not always want one's origins predetermined. On the contrary, where the presumption is in favour of variability and keeping a range of possibilities open, *anticipation could be disabling*. An alternative conclusion is that once we know all the available options, we can act.

Two different values are put on anticipation, then. The reproduction of recognisable forms implies a continuous identity. It is a type of anthropology that continues to unfold in Ortner's view, even as the outcome of embryonic growth should be a child with human features. Because of the predictability of outcome here, one can anticipate the result, a (new) anthropology or a (new) child, to whose fruition each stage of development contributes. Yet it is equally important that the result should be unique. The new anthropology really must be new, and one baby should not be exactly like another. The child's guarantee of individuality lies in genetic origin: its characteristics are the outcome of a chance combination from a range of possibilities. In the same way, the competing theories of different anthropologies in the past provide the potential for new combinations in the future. Defining one stage by what it will become thus anticipates a predictable future by virtue of its continuity with the present. Genetic potential, however, maintains an array of possible characteristics from which an entity might emerge; the future is known instead by its unpredictability, and one would not necessarily wish to anticipate it.

Now there is no simple alignment of concepts here. In encompassing they also reproduce one another, though exemplification will inevitably depend on one's starting point and the links one values. Thus a relation between heredity and development can be replicated in terms internal to each, since either may be held to demonstrate change and continuity; change in turn may be understood as comprising either an episodic or an evolutionary view of time, and so forth. It might seem gratuitous to introduce the further difference between the values put on anticipation, but I do so for specific effect.

The proliferation and apparent cross-overs in ideas provide grounds for fertile debate. But the practice of debate requires that critical decisions are made. Indeed, taking a position activates the very potential that lies in knowledge, that if we know where we are or what our options are, we can act. It is of interest therefore to consider a public debate that has been concerned with establishing just such preconditions to action, and with reference to new possibilities in human reproduction. Much of the debate occurred in anticipation of the 1990 Human Fertilisation and Embryology Act.

I dwell briefly on certain issues raised in connection with the status of the human embryo. Advances in reproductive medicine that have enabled fertilised eggs to be produced outside the body, and available for experimentation, necessitated legislation on the status of such material/beings. The parliamentary deliberation culminated in a decision to make one particular stage in the process of embryonic development a definitive divide. This was at 14 days' growth, just prior to the emergence of the 'primitive streak' which signalled the presence of an individual entity. Before then any of a number of futures was possible; after that point, whatever else happened, if the entity were to develop at all it would have a singular identity. In the words of a non-parliamentary commentator, 'once the primitive streak is established, so is individuality' (Dunstan 1990: 6; cf. Fagot-Largeault 1990: 152).*

The larger public debate found itself directly addressing the relationship between developmental process and the identity bestowed by heredity origin. It is not surprising to find a concomitant engagement with change and continuity. What is also of interest is that, in the treatment of origins, it is the origins of an entity's individuality which proved crucial, and that the concept of individuality was understood in a social or 'metaphysical' sense as well as a 'biological' one (Solbaak 1990: 103). Indeed, we might expect the language to evoke ways of thinking about procreation that are found also in kinship constructs and ideas about relations between persons and thus in the reproductive model. After all, if the reproductive model informs how people may think about the future, as a model of the future it may also inform how they may think about reproduction.

Potentiality

In a phrase that echoes Ortner's, Warnock observed in 1987 that 'how far they are along the road' will enable us to understand 'what they are'. Harris (1990: 72) quotes the statement in a discussion about experiments on embryos. 'They' are gametes and the trend is towards their 'becoming fully human'.[12]

Heredity concerns not just kinship identity or the transmission of individual characteristics, but the very origin of human substance in human substance. At the same time, living human beings exist only as persons, and in the Euro-American view this means as conscious individual subjects. In the context of these debates individuality is construed as an outcome of organic development. The significance of individuality and the facts of developmental process are taken for granted; the debate tries to establish the fact of individuality through the significance of the developmental stage. For since development is popularly held to be continuous rather

---

* An issue raised at the beginning of this volume (see Chapter 1). I do not discuss the reasons why such a divide was sought, only the already existing (cultural) concepts that led to the formula of 'individuality'.

than catastrophic, the principal problem seems to lie in determining what stage an entity has reached.

This, in part, is how such matters were aired at the 1988 Conference on Philosophical Ethics in Reproductive Medicine (PERM) (Bromham, *et al.* 1990). Since actions will affect the future of the organism, it is necessary to know what one is dealing with. Different consequences flow from conceiving an entity as living cells, as human substance or as a person-to-be, for different values are put on life, humanness and personhood. Determining the stage the organism has reached thus offers it a future. But the very act of anticipation raises a problem: several speakers addressed the questionable difference between potential as opposed to actual identity. The question is presupposed in imagining the relation between past and future in terms of origins and links.

At first blush, it looks as though exponents[13] divide into holders of evolutionary and episodic views of time. Those who speak from the view of process may draw biology into their representation of development as continuous. Others take certain moments as radical beginnings, notably those who maintain that the conceptus exists from 'the moment' of fertilisation.[14] Yet each position also encompasses the other. Thus the evolutionary view requires that stages be demarcated in accord with specific social constructions put on their significance − for example, the definitive point at which sentience is evident; while the episodic view may defend the pre-existence of the conceptus because of its destiny as a human being − even if to the scientific probe it is not clear which of a set of cells will develop into a person, all should be protected because of those that will. Each thus appropriates facts also acknowledged by the other side. Hence it is possible to shift an evolutionary argument with respect to what something might become into an episodic argument that tries to avoid any anticipatory effect in favour of an unpredictable future.

While some argue that the simple fact of cells being alive warrants no special treatment, that gametes are human cells of a particular kind gives others pause. Their own reproductive potential seems significant. (We might call this an ideational potential; their 'actual' potential changes with their stage of development (cf. Birke *et al.* 1990: 70).) Cells are routinely shed by the body or removed by surgery, but here a link with the future is anticipated. For in these particular ones lie the origins of human beings: all they seemingly require is fertilisation and implantation. Now since human beings exist in actuality as singular entities, in the Euro-American view, it is possible to argue that an 'actual' human being is not discernible until individuality also is — however early or late this is deemed to be evident. Individuality in turn comes to have an origin; individuation as a developmental stage makes it further possible to attribute 'moral force to the principle ... that protection due is related to morphological growth' (Dunstan 1990: 5).

Dunstan, 'matching protection to growth, to progress towards maturity', evokes the thought that 'there can be no human personality without individuality' (1990: 6).[15] This must anticipate the social meaning of individuation: indeed he adds, 'without individuality there can be no moral agency, no accountability, no identity' (1990: 6). For the stage in question, it is not that the clump of cells at one end of the embryonic disc, which indicates the emergence of the primitive streak, has moral agency, but that the streak marks the starting point of an entity whose only future is as an individual and which thus meets the first condition of this (Euro-American) view of personhood. In effect, Dunstan implies that this is *the actual establishment of a significant potential*. The value put on anticipation could go either way at this point.

Dunstan draws a non-anticipatory conclusion. He takes the philosophical position that one cannot argue back from what might have been (the potentiality thesis), so there is no absolute duty to protect the embryo even after the primitive streak appears. Rather, he concludes that the possibility of intervention in the early stages of development has made out of the human embryo a distinctive object of knowledge and moral attention for what it is (the actuality thesis).

In this latter view, the 'human embryo' now exists as a new object of thought in the world. It will require new ways of thinking and regulative practices specific to it, regardless of where it has come from or where it is going. That it has come from human cells is not definitive, for it requires subsequent morphological development to turn into an individual embryo; that it may become a person is irrelevant, for it is not yet at that stage. As for Warnock (1985: 60), the question is 'how it is right to treat the human embryo' as such. But to avoid the potentiality argument, moral significance must be decided (episodically) 'in terms of what they [the gametes] are at the particular moment at which the judgement is made'

(Harris 1990: 72).[16] Harris himself belittles the potentiality thesis by declaring: 'we are all potentially dead, but no-one supposes that this fact constitutes a reason for treating us as if we were already dead' (1990: 70).

This evokes a Melanesian reflection. Treating one as though one were already dead seems just the effect for which the people of Tanga strive when they envisage the immortality of the (matri)lineage. In other Melanesian societies, the elderly may even anticipate death to the point of demanding pre-mortem sacrifice. Now death is as much a certainty for Euro-Americans as for Melanesians. But the former maintain that the manner should be unpredictable, and that dying is impossible to bring forward without murderous or military intent. One attends to the present because the condition of the living person is not that of a deceased. In addition, one does not want to know how death will come; to anticipate would threaten the hope that is contained within the chanciness of when it will happen.

Chance also enters the discussions about life. Warnock (1985: 60) traces the beginning of the moral debate over embryos to those programmes for *in vitro* fertilisation that 'gave rise to the possibility that human embryos might be brought into existence which might have no chance to implant because they were not transferred to a uterus and hence no chance to be born as human beings'. This almost implies that each embryonic stage should be protected in order to give chance itself a chance. One does not anticipate the (statistical) likelihood of non-survival for that would preempt chance itself. Such an anticipation would indeed be disabling.

Potentiation and disablement

Does the potentiality debate help anthropologists think about where their subject is going?

Suppose the subject did have the potential to develop into something else, how would that effect what we do at present? Would we claim to have seeded the future? Or would we prefer to keep options open, even allowing for imperfections in ways of thinking if by analogy with genetic variation imperfections become 'the source of the individual variation we so much prize in ourselves' (Grobstein 1990: 16)? Or do we take reflection on what should be protected as creating – like the human embryo – a new object of knowledge in itself (cf. Thornton 1991)? Or is it the reproductive model that is the problem? Perhaps it makes us greedy for both change and continuity, as though one could bring about momentous (episodic) change while still being regarded as the continuous (evolutionary) originators of it. This seems not to be a problem for Melanesians in the ethnographic literature: for them, the future is premised on discontinuity.

But those 'Melanesians', what are they but orientalised objects of anthropological knowledge, out of date even as they were written about? In any case, 'their' traditions are vanishing. And 'ours' are not?

It looks as though those troublesome kinship constructs, manifest in the Euro-American reproductive model of change and continuity, will not trouble us for much longer. We can relegate them to some distant modernist epoch when the human quest included the search for links and origins and led to questions about where one was going. It is the search that has done it; Schneider (1968: 23) once said that whatever scientists found out about biogenetic relationship would be taken as knowledge about kinship, and his prophecy seems to have come true with respect to the reproductive model. Except that I wonder if the result will be kinship.

Ever since genetics informed popular knowledge about the transmission of characteristics, it has been taken as special evidence for the chanciness of individual endowment. Chancy origins thus match chancy futures, for individuals also vary by their fortunes in life. At the same time, genetic transmission miniaturises the reproductive model. It encompasses or contains within itself a differentiation constitutive of the model as such: a relation between what is (heredity leading to developmental fruition) and what is not (heredity as random variation) appropriately anticipated. Yet that containment of differentiation has in the recent past depended on the particular place that ideas about genetic transmission occupied in the model as a whole, as the signifier of the chancy outcome as opposed to the inevitable, planned one. The interesting question is what happens when knowledge about the genetic composition of persons turns the miniature into the whole. For the significance of genetic origins and links is taking an increasing hold in adjudications about procreative possibilities (and see Franklin 1991).* I do not mean that biologists would

---

* This is the point at which to thank two participants of the 1990 Association for Social Anthropology Conference for comments which inspired the writing of the present essay: Vered Talai's observations on the geneticisation of kin identity and David Parkin's taking my apprehensiveness seriously.

ever overlook developmental or environmental contingencies. I refer rather to the way the potential of genetic identification has created a new object of popular knowledge *for conceptualising persons*: genetic destiny.

The possibilities of certainty have here created a new focus of moral attention. Thus the 'genetic parent' has become party to adjudications about rights and responsibilities. In the case of a woman having an embryo or gametes placed in her, the explanatory memorandum to the then Human Embryology and Fertilisation Bill qualified its definition of motherhood by reference to the child being genetically hers or not. There are also new implications to transmission. In the case of a person conceived by donor insemination, it was recommended that information about the donor's origin be disclosable on the grounds of 'genetic health' (see Snowden 1990: 81), a new consideration in the way children might think about parents.

Perhaps the current interest in genetic origins will turn out to have been more of a radical (episodic) break with the past, and with the old reproductive model, than it is an (evolutionary) development of what we already know. All those questions about location, identity and the road ahead become collapsible into knowledge about genetic destiny. I am not so certain that we shall in the future need representations of downward inheritance or of relations embodied in relationships: all we shall need is the programme itself. The *idea* of a programme obviates the idea of chance. Questions that the individual person once asked of him- or herself about origin and links need no longer be asked of kinship when they can be asked of the individual's genome.

In talking about manipulation and experiment, Grobstein makes a strong argument for reminding ourselves that the human genome (the totality of hereditary material) is the collective property of humanity. The isue is too momentous: 'deliberate intervention should never occur without collective deliberation' (1990: 20). But how is the collectivity imagined? He appeals to *ideas of kinship*. While every individual human being has a unique genome, he argues, each such genome is best thought of 'as a node in an overall heredity web. Linking the nodes within the web there are kin relationships among members of a generation and also between succeeding generations' (1990: 20). So what kind of 'kinship' is this? Such a generalised community might care much about the pool but its only interest in the origins of specific links seems to concern 'the implications of gene transfer to germ-line cells' (1990: 20). It is the very idea of genetic destiny that puts 'kinship' at risk.

Biologists may rightly pour scorn on the idea that human variation is at any risk from the present potential to manipulate the gene pool (e.g. Ferguson 1990: 9). The genetic transmission of characteristics must remain for the most part a chancy affair. But what will remain of the model that puts value on chanciness and unpredictability? The thought of knowing the combination of characteristics one is endowed with offers anticipation of a new kind. Thus advances in genetic knowledge ('mapping the genome') may well put us in the position of treating persons, if not as though they were dead, then at least in terms of what diseases they are likely to die of. It is popularly held that this will be knowledge on which bureaucracies will want to act.

As part of a project to increase public awareness of the role biotechnology plays in twentieth-century society, Yoxen (1983: 240) several years ago argued for a study of the future. He had in mind the 'culturing' of possible futures to imagine what they would be like. 'The hope is that we would learn to adopt a less passive attitude towards innovation and start, first, to interrogate technical experts in a more confident way, and then to participate in the process of designing the future.' It is not quite certain which culture would provide a model for culturing. But it does seem that his designed futures are neither millenarian nor utopian. They are rather what we must do to equally take advantage and mitigate against the disadvantages of developments whose effects are already present.

It was once the case that the idea of new combinations of genes producing vigorous hybrids, sources of innovation and originality, symbolised the power of the unpredictable. But if the genetic origin/ link is nowadays 'real' kinship, and if a genetic programme is popularly thought to have its own momentum, then will the rest of human affairs − relationships, events, cultures − be seen as a surrogate for reality? Against too much design, shall we find ourselves hoping not for the planned outcomes but for the chancy ones? To appreciate 'nature' not for the predictability of its laws but for the saving grace of the butterfly effect? And on the side of chance, shall we also put those social regularities and cultural norms that anthropologists once took to represent the predictable in human history? What then should anthropology reproduce?

I have implied that many anthropological habits of thought are as continuous with the folk models of the society to which they belong as they are discontinuous from models anthropologists encounter elsewhere. But that carries its own rider. My Melanesian examples have been drawn from diverse sources in place and time. It is irrelevant to the present account (but certainly not to understanding Melanesia) whether the practices I describe survive today. For it cannot be the disappearance of Melanesian customs that will change the future of anthropology; they were always objects and in that sense creations of anthropological knowledge. The disappearance of Euro-American customs, however, is another matter. The vanishing of taken-for-granted assumptions about natural process, about continuity and change, and about individuality, will make the future for us. Quite how we shall operate the reproductive model will be of some moment. Melanesia may or may not come to look 'other' in the process.

Notes

1 These are the terms in which components of biological knowledge are 'translated' for a non-expert audience.

2 The particular emphasis put on the role of parenting in assisting the *development* of the child as an individual entity is a distinctive feature of English (and Western) kin constructs. Franklin (1991) discusses common images of the relationship between development and the teleology attributed to genetic 'determinism'.

3 Whether through the idea of the unfolding of a pre-formed shape or through the active creation of form through differentiation from a previously unformed mass. In ways of thinking about embryo development, the first (preformationism) has historically been displaced by the second (epigenesis) (Birke *et al.* 1990: 69–70). However, the first remains tenacious in popular thinking. I present one version of it below in arguments about potentiality.

4 The permutations entailed in such perception of change and continuity are manifold. The model is constituted in the way each of its parts (or applications) replicates the analogies that hold the whole.

5 One version of such calibration lies in contrasts between sexual and asexual renewal (Foster 1990: 434); in the example he cites the former entailing (episodic) birth and death, the latter the ('evolutionary') shedding of skins. Plant growth provides metaphors of gradual transformation in numerous contexts.

6 A pervasive theme in the literature on the Eastern Highlands (e.g. Gillison 1980), from which I draw the archetype. For an overview, see Hays (1986) and the discussions in Gewertz (1988).

7 'Women' are frequently said to be the cause of fights or disputes. The fact does not make women important. Rather what is signified is the triviality of the originating cause, true of the most momentous of events – the bringing of death into the world or clans engaged in prolonged hostilities. The point is that what triggered such actions off is *displaced* by what follows, and is not necessarily retrospectively aggrandised. I thank Matthew McKeown for his insights here.

8 The Mandak of New Ireland hold mortuary feasts to 'finish all talk' about the deceased, who must be dispatched as social beings (the 'talk' that surrounds people signifies their effect on the world). For a critical discussion see Battaglia (1990: 196); she refers to Sabarl Island mortuary ritual as mimicking death by stopping the future flow of memories from having further creative effect.

9 Foster (1990: 438) emphasises the coercive nature of the relationship. They consume the analogue to what was once the product of their own bodies; in this reassimilation of substance they take back what they earlier transmitted, a kind of reverse inheritance. (Indeed, rather than distributing it, the survivors gather up everything that the deceased received in his or her lifetime and turn it into non-distributable matrilineage property.)

10 'Understanding how society and culture themselves are produced and reproduced through human intention and action' (Ortner 1984: 158). Needless to say, Melanesian models produce and reproduce persons and relationships; 'society' is not an object of their procreative effort, nor is 'anthropology' for that matter.

11 True whether the intellectual intention is to overthrow or sustain past values. Self-conscious 'breaks' with the past may well include painstaking attempts to define the inevitability of the present moment.

12 Warnock (1987: 8) is quoted as saying: 'To say that eggs and sperm cannot by themselves become human, but only if bound together, does not seem to me to differentiate them from the early embryo which by itself will not become human either, but will die unless it is implanted'.

13 I refer to positions discussed at the conference, not necessarily to ones that the speakers occupied. Of the contributors whom I cite, the Revd Gordon Dunstan offers a view from moral theology; Clifford Grobstein is an American embryologist by training; Peter Singer is Director of a Centre for Human Bioethics in Australia; Robert Snowden is a Professor of Family Studies. The references to Harris, Ferguson and Warnock are to other publications.

14 There is no 'moment' of fertilisation, biologically speaking, any more than development is regarded as a simple unfolding (see note 3). But the debate in general was constructed in terms of an opposition between continuity and discontinuity.*

* My argument is guided by the direction that the PERM Conference took; for a view on the idea that human beings are present from the start of embryonic life see the citation of Holland by Morgan and Lee (1991: 70–71).

15 'Boethius is quoted down the centuries ... a person is an individual partaking in rational nature. And rational nature is, of course, the common property of humanity. An *individual* there must be, to become eventually the bearer of rights, the embodiment of human attributes and agency' (Dunstan 1990: 6, original emphasis).

16 An argument for considering the present state of the embryo rather than a future one, not an argument for deriving morality from biology. Singer's (1990: 38) observation would be widely shared: 'To settle factual or definitional questions about the beginning of a new biological life is not to settle the moral question of how we should treat such biologically defined entities'. He himself observes that just as a warm, living body needs no protection for its own sake once its brain is destroyed, so an embryo needs no protection till its brain has developed into a functioning organism. Compare Warnock's statement above [p. 173]. Harris, in effect, points out that Warnock moves between episodic (actuality) and evolutionary (potentiality) arguments.

REFERENCES

Abrahams, R. (1990), 'Plus ça change, plus c'est la même chose?', *The Australian Journal of Anthropology*, special issue [Essays in honour of John Barnes], 1, 131–46.

Alcoff, L. (1988), 'Cultural feminism versus post-structuralism: the identity crisis in feminist theory', *Signs*, 13, 405–36.

Barnett, S. and Magdoff, J. (1986), 'Beyond narcissism in American culture of the 1980s', *Cultural Anthropology*, 1, 413–24.

Battaglia, D. (1985), ' "We feed our father": paternal nurture among the Sabarl of Papua New Guinea', *American Ethnologist*, 12, 427–41.

Battaglia, D. (1990), *On the Bones of the Serpent: Person, Memory and Mortality in Sabarl Island Society*, University of Chicago Press, Chicago.

Battaglia, D. (1991), 'Punishing the yams: leadership and gender ambivalence on Sabarl'. In M. Godelier and M. Strathern (eds), *Big Men and Great Men. Personifications of Power in Melanesia*, Cambridge University Press, Cambridge.

Beer, G. (1983), *Darwin's Plots. Evolutionary Narrative in Darwin, George Eliot and Nineteenth Century Fiction*, Routledge and Kegan Paul, London.

Best, S. (1991), 'Chaos and entropy: metaphors in postmodern science and social theory', *Science as Culture*, 11, 188–226.

Biagioli, M. (1990), 'Galileo's system of patronage', *History of Science*, 28, 1–62.

Biersack, A. (1982), 'Ginger gardens for the ginger woman: rites and passages in a Melanesian society', *Man* (N.S.), 17, 239–58.

Birke, L., Himmelweit, S. and Vines, G. (1990), *Tomorrow's Child: Reproductive Technologies in the 90s*, Virago, London.

Bloch, M. (1986), *From Blessing to Violence. History and Ideology in the Circumcision Ritual of the Merina of Madagascar*, Cambridge University Press, Cambridge.

Blowers, A., Hamnett, C. and Sarre, P. (eds) (1974), *The Future of Cities*, Hutchinson Educational, London.

Bonnemère, P. (n.d.), 'Constitution and treatment of the human body among the Ankave-Anga of Papua New Guinea: the making of a bilateral sociality'. Paper delivered to 2nd Melanesian Colloquium, *Embodiment and Sociality*, Manchester, 1991.

Boon, J.A. (1982), *Other Tribes, Other Scribes. Symbolic Anthropology in the Comparative Study of Cultures, Histories, Religions, and Texts*, Cambridge University Press, Cambridge.

Braidotti, R. (1988), 'Organs without bodies', *Differences: A Journal of Feminist Cultural Studies*, 1, 147–61.

Bromham, D. R., Dalton, M. E. and Jackson, J. C. (eds) (1990), *Philosophical Ethics in Reproductive Medicine*, Manchester University Press, Manchester.

Buckley, T. and Gottlieb, A. (1988), *Blood Magic. The Anthropology of Menstruation*, University of California Press, Berkeley & Los Angeles.

Cannell, F. (1990), 'Concepts of parenthood: the Warnock Report, the Gullick debate, and modern myths', *American Ethnologist*, 17, 667–86.

Caplan, P. (ed.) (1987), *The Cultural Construction of Sexuality*, Tavistock, London.

Carrier, J. (n.d.), 'Cultural content and practical meaning: the construction of symbols in formal American culture', ms, Port Moreby, Papua New Guinea.

Cheal, D. (1988), *The Gift Economy*, Routledge, London.

Chowning, A. (1989), 'Death and kinship in Molima'. In F. Damon and R. Wagner (eds), *Death Rituals and Life in the Societies of the Kula Ring*, Northern Illinois University Press, De Kalb.

Clark, J. (1991), 'Pearlshell symbolism in Highland Papua New Guinea, with particular reference to the Wiru people of Southern Highlands Province', *Oceania*, 61: 309–39.

Clay, B. J. (1986), *Mandak Realities: Person and Power in Central New Ireland*, Rutgers University Press, New Brunswick, NJ.

Clifford, J. (1986), 'Partial truths', Introduction to *Writing Culture*, J. Clifford and G. E. Marcus (eds), University of California Press, Berkeley & Los Angeles.

Clifford, J. (1988), *The Predicament of Culture: Twentieth Century Ethnography, Literature, and Art*, Harvard University Press, Cambridge, Mass.

Clifford, J. and Marcus, G. E. (eds) (1986), *Writing Culture: The Poetics and Politics of Ethnography*, University of California Press, Berkeley & Los Angeles.

Cohen, A. P. (1987), *Whalsay. Symbol, Segment and Boundary in a Shetland Island Community*, Manchester University Press, Manchester.

Coppet, D. de (1981), 'The life-giving death'. In S. C. Humphreys and H. King (eds), *Mortality and Immortality: The Anthropology and Archaeology of Death*, Academic Press, London.

Coppet, D. de (1985), 'Land owns people'. In R. H. Barnes, D. de Coppet and R. J. Parkin (eds), *Contexts and Levels. Anthropological Essays on Hierarchy*, JASO, Oxford.

Culler, J. (1979), 'Jaques Derrida'. In J. Sturrock (ed.), *Structuralism and Since*, Oxford University Press, Oxford.

Dalton, G. (1990), 'The moral status of the human embryo'. In D. Bromham, M. E. Dalton and J. C. Jackson (eds), *Philosophical Ethics in Reproductive Medicine*, Manchester University Press, Manchester.

Damon, F. (1989), 'The Muyuw *lo'un* and the end of marriage'. In F. Damon and R. Wagner (eds), *Death Rituals and Life in the Societies of the Kula Ring*, Northern Illinois University Press, De Kalb.

Damon, F. and Wagner, R. (eds) (1989), *Death Rituals and Life in the Societies in the Kula Ring*, Northern Illinois University Press, De Kalb.

Davidoff, L. and Hall, C. (1987), *Family Fortunes. Men and Women of the English Middle Class 1780–1850*, Hutchinson, London.

Davis, N. Z. (n.d.), 'Gifts, markets and communities in sixteenth century France'. Presented to conference *The Gift and its Transformations*, National Humanities Center, North Carolina, 1990.

di Leonardo, M. (1985), 'Deindustrialization as a folk model', *Urban Anthropology*, 14, 237–57.

Dolgin, J. L. (1990), 'Status and contract in surrogate motherhood: an illumination of the surrogacy debate', *Buffalo Law Review*, 38, 515–50.

Dunstan, G. (1990), 'The moral status of the human embryo'. In D. R. Bromham, M. E. Dalton and J. C. Jackson (eds), *Philosophical Ethics in Reproductive Medicine*, Manchester University Press, Manchester.

Dyson, A. (1990), 'At Heaven's command?: the churches, theology and experiments on embryos'. In A. Dyson and J. Harris (eds), *Experiments on Embryos*, Routledge, London.

Fagot-Largeault, A. (1990), 'The notion of the potential human being'. In D. R. Bromham, M. E. Dalton and J. C. Jackson (eds), *Philosophical Ethics in Reproductive Medicine*, Manchester University Press, Manchester.

Feher, M. with R. Nadaff and N. Tazi (1989), *Fragments for a History of the Human Body*, 3 vols., Zone [MIT Press], New York.

Ferguson, M. W. J. (1990), 'Contemporary and future possibilities for human embryonic manipulation'. In A. Dyson and J. Harris (eds), *Experiments on Embryos*, Routledge, London.

Finch, J. (1989), *Family Obligations and Social Change*, Polity Press, Oxford.

Firth, R. and Djamour, J. (1956), 'Kinship in South Borough'. In F. Firth (ed.), *Two Studies of Kinship in London*, Athlone Press, London.

Firth, R., Hubert, J. and Forge, A. (1969), *Families and their Relatives. Kinship in a Middle-Class Sector of London*, Routledge and Kegal Paul, London.

Fisher, M. M. J., Marcus, G. and Tyler, S. A. (1988), Response to Sangren, 'Rhetoric and the authority of anthropology', *Current Anthropology*, 29, 425–6.

Fortes, M. (1958), Introduction to J. Goody (ed.), *The Developmental Cycle in Domestic Groups*, Cambridge University Press, Cambridge.

Fortes, M. (1969), *Kinship and the Social Order*, Aldine, Chicago.

Fortes, M. (1970), *Time and Social Structure, and Other Essays*, Athlone Press, London.

Fortes, M. (1984), Foreword to P. Lawrence, *The Garia*, Melbourne University Press, Melbourne.

Foster, R. (1990), 'Nurture and force-feeding: mortuary feasting and the construction of collective individuals in a New Ireland society', *American Ethnologist*, 17, 431−48.

Fox, R. (1967), *Kinship and Marriage. An Anthropological Perspective*, Penguin, London.

Franklin, S. (1991), 'Fetal fascinations: the construction of fetal personhood and the Alton debate'. In S. Franklin, C. Lury and J. Stacey (eds), *Off-Centre: Feminism and Cultural Studies*, Unwin Hyman, London.

Franklin, S. (n.d.), 'Making sense of missed conceptions: anthropological perspectives on unexplained fertility'. Paper presented to 152nd Annual Meeting, *British Association for the Advancement of Science*, Swansea, 1990.

Franklin, S. and McNeill, M. (1988), 'Review essay: recent literature and current feminist debates on reproductive technologies', *Feminist Studies*, 14, 545−60.

Freeman, D. (1961), 'On the concept of the kindred', *Journal of Royal Anthropological Institute*, 91, 192−220.

Gallagher, J. (1987), 'Eggs, embryos and foetuses: anxiety and the law'. In M. Stanworth (ed.), *Reproductive Technologies*, Polity Press, Oxford.

Geertz, C. (1973), *The Interpretation of Cultures*, Basic Books, New York.

Gellner, E. (1964), *Thought and Change*, University of Chicago Press, Chicago.

Gewertz, D. (ed.) (1988), *Myths of Matriarchy Reconsidered*, University of Sydney, Oceania Monograph 33.

Giddens, A. (1984), *The Constitution of Society*, Polity Press, Oxford.

Gillison, G. (1980), 'Images of nature in Gimi thought'. In C. MacCormack and M. Strathern (eds), *Nature, Culture and Gender*, Cambridge University Press, Cambridge.

Gillison, G. (1987), 'Incest and the atom of kinship: the role of the mother's brother in a New Guinea Highlands society', *Ethos*, 15, 166−202.

Gillison, G. (1991), 'The flute myth and the law of equivalence: origins of a principle of exchange'. In M. Godelier and M. Strathern (eds), *Big Men and Great Men. Personifications of Power in Melanesia*, Cambridge University Press, Cambridge.

Ginsburg, F. (1987), 'Procreation stories: reproduction, nurturance and procreation in life narratives of abortion activists', *American Ethnologist*, 14, 623−36.

Gleick, J. (1987), *Chaos: Making a New Science*, Heinemann, London.

Glover, J. *et al.* (1989), *Fertility and the Family*. The Glover Report on Reproductive Technologies to the European Commission, Fourth Estate, London.

Godelier, M. (1986) (trans. R. Swyer [1982]), *The Making of Great Men. Male Domination and Power among the New Guinea Baruya*, Cambridge University Press, Cambridge.

Godelier, M. (n.d.), 'Bodies, kinship and powers in the Baruya culture (Papua New Guinea)'. Paper delivered to 2nd Melanesian Colloquium, *Embodiment and Sociality*, Manchester, 1991.

Gregory, C.A. (1980), 'Gifts to men and gifts to God: gift exchange and capital accumulation in contemporary Papua', *Man* (N.S.), 15, 626–52.

Gregory, C.A. (1982), *Gifts and Commodities*, Academic Press, London.

Grobstein, C. (1990), 'Genetic manipulation and experimentation'. In D.R. Bromham, M.E. Dalton and J.C. Jackson (eds), *Philosophical Ethics in Reproductive Medicine*, Manchester University Press, Manchester.

Haimes, E. (n.d.), 'Gender, gametes and the new reproductive technologies'. Paper given to BSA Annual Conference, Manchester, 1991.

Hannerz, U. (1988), 'American culture: creolized, creolizing'. In E. Åsard (ed.), *American Culture: Creolized, Creolizing and other lectures from the NAAS Biennial Conference in Uppsala, May 28–31, 1987*, Swedish Institute for North American Studies, Uppsala.

Hannerz, U. (1990), 'Cosmopolitans and locals in world culture', *Theory, Culture and Society*, 7, 211–25.

Hannerz, U. (in press), 'The cultural role of world cities'. In A. Cohen and K. Fukui (eds), *The Age of the City*, Edinburgh University Press, Edinburgh.

Haraway, D. (1988), 'Situated knowledges: the science question in feminism as a site of discourse on the privilege of partial perspective', *Feminist Studies*, 14, 575–99.

Harding, S. (1986), 'The instability of the analytical categories of feminist theory', *Signs: Journal of Women in Culture and Society*, 11, 645–64.

Harris, J. (1990), 'Embryos and hedgehogs: on the moral status of the embryo'. In A. Dyson and J. Harris (eds), *Experiments on Embryos*, Routledge, London.

Harrison, S. (1985), 'Concepts of the person in Avatip religious thought', *Man* (N.S.), 20, 115–30.

Hayles, N.K. (1990), 'Designs on the body: Norbert Weiner, cybernetics and the play of metaphor', *History of the Human Sciences*, 3, 211–28.

Hays, T.E. (1986), 'Sacred flutes, fertility, and growth in the Papua New Guinea Highlands', *Anthropos*, 81, 435–53.

HMSO (1987), *Human Fertilisation and Embryology: A Framework for Legislation*, Department of Health and Social Security, London.

Houseman, M. (1988), 'Towards a complex model of parenthood: two African tales', *American Ethnologist*, 15, 658–77.

Howard, A. (1988), 'Hypermedia and the future of anthropology', *Cultural Anthropology*, 3, 304–15.

Ingold, T. (1986), *Evolution and Social Life*, Cambridge University Press, Cambridge.

Ingold, T. (1988), 'Tools, minds and machines: an excursion in the philosophy of technology', *Techniques et culture*, 12, 151–76.

Ingold, T. (n.d.), 'Culture and the perception of the envirionment'. For workshop on *Cultural Understandings of the Environment*, School of Oriental and African Studies, London, 1989.

Iteanu, A. (1990), 'The concept of the person and the ritual system: an Orokaiva view', *Man* (N.S.), 25, 35–53.

Jencks, C. [and Keswick, M.] (1987), *What is Post Modernism?*, Academy Editions, London/St. Martin's Press, New York [2nd edn].

Johnson, M. (1989), 'Did I begin?', *New Scientist*, 9 December, 39–42.

Jordanova, L. (1980), 'Natural facts: a historical perspective on science and sexuality'. In C. MaCormack and M. Strathern (eds), *Nature, Culture and Gender*, Cambridge University Press, Cambridge.

Josephides, L. (1985), *The Production of Inequality. Gender and Exchange among the Kewa*, Tavistock, London.

Keat, R. (1990), 'Starship Britain or universal enterprise'. In R. Keat and N. Abercrombie (eds), *Enterprise Culture*, Routledge, London.

Kirby, V. (1989), 'Capitalizing difference: feminism and anthropology', *Australian Feminist Studies*, 9, 1–24.

Klein, R. D. (ed.) (1989), *Infertility*, Pandora Press, London.

Kuper, A. (1982), 'Lineage theory: a critical retrospect', *Annual Reviews of Anthropology*, 11, 71–95.

Kuper, A. (1988), *The Invention of Primitive Society. Transformations of an Illusion*, Routledge, London.

Lattas, A. (n.d.), 'Sacrifice, tambarans and the appropriation of female reproductive powers in male initiation ceremonies in West New Britain', ms, Adelaide.

Lawrence, P. (1969), 'The state versus stateless societies in Papua New Guinea'. In B. J. Brown (ed.), *Fashion of Law in New Guinea*, Butterworth, Sydney.

Lawrence, P. (1971), 'The Garia of the Madang District'. In R. M. Berndt and P. Lawrence (eds), *Politics in New Guinea*, University of Western Australia Press, Nedlands.

Lawrence, P. (1984), *The Garia. An Ethnography of a Traditional Cosmic System in Papua New Guinea*, Melbourne University Press, Melbourne.

Lederman, R. (1986), *What Gifts Engender: Social Relations and Politics in Mendi, Highland Papua New Guinea*, Cambridge University Press, Cambridge.

Leenhardt, M. (1979) [1947], *Do Kamo. Person and Myth in the Melanesian World* (trans. B. M. Gulati), University of Chicago Press, Chicago.

Leicester, C. (1974) [1970], 'Life in the year AD 2000'. In A. Blowers, C. Hamnet and P. Sarre (eds), *The Future of Cities*, Hutchinson Educational, London.

Lévi, J. (1989), 'The body: the Daoists' coat of arms'. In M. Feher *et al.*, *Fragments for a History of the Human Body*, Zone [MIT Press], New York.

Lévi-Strauss, C. (1955), *Tristes tropiques*, Plon, Paris.

Lowenthal, D. (1990), 'Awareness of human impacts: changing attitudes and emphases'. In B. L. Turner (ed.), *Earth Transformed*, Cambridge University Press, Cambridge.

McDowell, N. (1985), 'Past and future: the nature of episodic time in Bun'. In D. Gewertz and E. Schieffelin (eds), *History and Ethnohistory in Papua New Guinea*, University of Sydney, Oceania Monograph 28.

Macfarlane, A. (1986), *Marriage and Love in England. Modes of Reproduction 1300–1840*, Basil Blackwell, Oxford.

Malamond, C. (1989), 'Indian speculations about the sex of the sacrifice'. In M. Feher *et al.*, *Frgments for a History of the Human Body*, Zone [MIT Press], New York.

Martin, E. (1987), *The Woman in the Body. A Cultural Analysis of Reproduction*, Beacon Press, Boston.

May, R. J. (ed.) (1982), *Micronationalist Movements in Papua New Guinea*, Australian National University, Department of Political and Social Change, Canberra, Monograph 1.

Miller, D. (1987), *Material Culture and Mass Consumption*, Basil Blackwell, Oxford.

Miller, D. (1988), 'Appropriating the state on the council estate', *Man* (N.S.), 23, 353–72.

Mimica, J. (1988), *Intimations of Infinity: The Cultural Meanings of the Iqwaye Counting System and Number*, Berg, Oxford.

Miyaji, M. (in press), 'Family and social networks in new urban situations: a comparative perspective'. In A. Cohen and K. Fukui (eds), *The Age of the City*, Edinburgh University Press, Edinburgh.

Moi, T. (1985), *Sexual/Textual Politics: Feminist Literary Theory*, Routledge, London.

Moore, H. (1988), *Feminism and Anthropology*, Polity Press, Oxford.

Morgan, D. and Lee, R. (1991), *Blackstone's Guide to the Human Fertilisation and Embryology Act 1990: Abortion and Embryo Research, the New Law*, Blackstone Press, London.

Morgan, L. M. (1989), 'When does life begin? A cross-cultural perspective on the personhood of fetuses and young children'. In E. and J. Prescott (eds), *Abortion Rights and Fetal 'Personhood'*, Centerline Press, Long Beach, Calif.

Mosko, M. (1983), 'Conception, de-conception and social structure in Bush Mekeo culture', *Mankind*, Special Issue, *Concepts of Conception: procreation ideologies in Papua New Guinea*, D. Jorgensen (ed.).

Mosko, M. (1985), *Quadripartite Structure. Categories, Relations and Homologies in Bush Mekeo Culture*, Cambridge University Press, Cambridge.

Mosko, M. (1989), 'The developmental cycle among public groups', *Man* (N.S.), 24, 470–84.

Munn, N.D. (1986), *The Fame of Gawa. A Symbolic Study of Value Transformation in a Massim (Papua New Guinea) Society*, Cambridge University Press, Cambridge.

Ortner, S.B. (1984), 'Theory in anthropology since the sixties', *Comparative Studies in Society and History*, 26, 126–66.

Ortner, S.B. and Whitehead, H. (eds) (1981), *Sexual Meanings. The Cultural Construction of Gender and Sexuality*, Cambridge University Press, Cambridge.

Pahl, R.E. (1964), 'Urbs in rure', *Geographical Papers*, London School of Economics and Political Science, London.

Panoff, M. (1970), 'Marcel Mauss's *The Gift* revisited', *Man* (N.S.), 5, 60–70.

Parkin, D. (1987), 'Comparison as the search for continuity'. In L. Holy (ed.), *Comparative Anthropology*, Basil Blackwell, Oxford.

Parry, J. (1986), '*The Gift*, the Indian gift and the "Indian gift"', *Man* (N.S.), 21, 453–73.

Parry, J. and Bloch, M. (1989), *Money and the Morality of Exchange*, Cambridge University Press, Cambridge.

Petchesky, R.P. (1987), 'Foetal images: the power of visual culture in the politics of reproduction'. In M. Stanworth (ed.), *Reproductive Technologies*, Polity Press, Oxford.

Pfeffer, N. (1987), 'Artificial insemination, in-vitro fertilisation and the stigma of infertility'. In M. Stanworth (ed.), *Reproductive Technologies*, Polity Press, Oxford.

Price, F. (1989), 'Establishing guidelines: regulation and the clinical management of infertility'. In R. Lee and D. Morgan (eds), *Birthrights: Law and Ethics at the Beginnings of Life*, Routledge, London.

Rabinow, P. (1988), Response to Sangren, 'Rhetoric and the authority of anthropology', *Current Anthropology*, 29, 429–30.

Rabinow, P. (1989), *French Modern. Norms and Forms of the Social Environment*, MIT Press, Cambridge, Mass.

Radcliffe-Brown, A.R. (1950), Introduction to A.R. Radcliffe-Brown and D. Forde (eds), *African Systems of Kinship and Marriage*, Oxford University Press, London.

Radcliffe-Brown, A.R. (1952), *Structure and Function in Primitive Society*, Cohen and West, London.

Radcliffe-Brown, A. R. and Forde, D. (eds) (1950), *African Systems of Kinship and Marriage*, Oxford University Press, London.

Rapport, N. (n.d.), 'Passage to Britain: a stereotypical view of coming home to the Old World from the New', ms, University of Manchester.

Rivière, P. (1985), 'Unscrambling parenthood: the Warnock Report', *Anthropology Today*, 4, 2–7.

Rose, N. (1991), 'Governing the enterprising self'. In P. Heelas and P. Morris (eds), *The Values of the Enterprise Culture – The Moral Debate*, Unwin Hyman, London.

Said, E. W. (1978), *Orientalism*, Routledge and Kegan Paul, London.

Sangren, S. P. (1988), 'Rhetoric and the authority of ethnography: "post modernism" and the social reproduction of texts', *Current Anthropology*, 29, 405–35.

Scheffler, H. W. (1985), 'Filiation and affiliation', *Man* (N.S.), 20, 1–21.

Schneider, D. M. (1968), *American Kinship: A Cultural Account*, Prentice-Hall, Englewood Cliffs, NJ.

Schneider, D. M. (1984), *A Critique of the Study of Kinship*, University of Michigan Press, Ann Arbor.

Seal, V. (1990), *Whose Choice? Working Class Women and the Control of Fertility*, Fortress Books, London.

Singer, P. (1990), 'IVF and Australian law'. In D. R. Bromham, M. E. Dalton and J. C. Jackson (eds), *Philosophical Ethics in Reproductive Medicine*, Manchester University Press, Manchester.

Sissa, G. (1989), 'Subtle bodies'. In M. Feher *et al.* (eds), *Fragments for a History of the Human Body*, Part 3, Zone [MIT Press], New York.

Smart, C. (1987), ' "There is of course the distinction created by nature": law and the problem of paternity'. In M. Stanworth (ed.), *Reproductive Technologies*, Polity Press, Oxford.

Smith, G. (1987), 'The crisis of fatherhood', *Free Associations*, 9, 72–90.

Snowden, R. (1990), 'The family and artificial reproduction'. In D. R. Bromham, M. E. Dalton and J. C. Jackson (eds), *Philosophical Ethics in Reproductive Medicine*, Manchester University Press, Manchester.

Solbaak, J. H. (1990) [Contribution to Proceedings]. In D. R. Bromham, M. E. Dalton and J. C. Jackson (eds), *Philosophical Ethics in Reproductive Medicine*, Manchester University Press, Manchester.

Spallone, P. and Steinberg, D. L. (eds) (1987), *Made to Order: The Myth of Reproductive and Genetic Progress*, Pergamon Press, Oxford.

Stanworth, M. (ed.) (1987), *Reproductive Technologies. Gender, Motherhood and Medicine*, Polity Press, Oxford.

Stolcke, V. (1986), 'New reproductive technologies – same old fatherhood', *Critique of Anthropology*, 6, 5–31.

Strathern, M. (1985a), 'Dislodging a world view: challenge and counter-challenge in the relationship between feminism and anthropology', *Australian Feminist Studies*, 1, 1–25.

Strathern, M. (1985b), 'Discovering social control', *Journal of Law and Society*, 12, 111–34.

Strathern, M. (1988), *The Gender of the Gift. Problems with Women and Problems with Society in Melanesia*, University of California Press, Berkeley & Los Angeles.

Strathern, M. (1991), *Partial Connections*, Association for Social Anthropology in Oceania special publication 3, Rowman and Littlefield, Savage, Md.

Strathern, M. (1992), *After Nature: English Kinship in the Late Twentieth Century*, Cambridge University Press, Cambridge.

Tabet, P. (1987), 'Imposed reproduction: maimed sexuality', *Feminist Issues*, 7, 3–31.

Thornton, R. (1988), 'The rhetoric of ethnographic holism', *Cultural Anthropology*, 3, 285–303.

Thornton, R. (1991), 'The end of the future?', Editorial, *Anthropology Today*, (7(1), 1–2.

Threadgold, T. (1988), 'Language and gender', *Australian Feminist Studies*, 6, 41–70.

Trautmann, T. R. (1987), *Lewis Henry Morgan and the Invention of Kinship*, University of California Press, Berkeley & Los Angeles.

Tuzin, D. F. (1982), 'Ritual violence among the Ilahita Arapesh'. In G. Herdt (ed.), *Rituals of Manhood*, University of California Press, Berkeley & Los Angeles.

Wagner, R. (1977), 'Analogic kinship: a Daribi example', *American Ethnologist*, 4, 623–42.

Wagner, R. (1986a), *Symbols that Stand for Themselves*, University of Chicago Press, Chicago.

Wagner, R. (1986b), *Asiwinarong: Ethos, Image, and Social Power among the Usen Barok of New Ireland*, Princeton University Press, Princeton, NJ.

Wagner, R. (1987), 'Daribi and Barok images of public man: a comparison'. In L. L. Langness and T. E. Hays (eds), *Anthropology in the High Valleys*, Chandler and Sharp, Novato, Calif.

Wagner, R. (1991), 'The fractal person'. In M. Godelier and M. Strathern (eds), *Big Men and Great Men. Personifications of Power in Melanesia*, Cambridge University Press, Cambridge.

Ward, K. (1990), 'An irresolvable dispute?' In A. Dyson and J. Harris (eds), *Experiments on Embryos*, Routledge, London.

Warnock, M. (1985), *A Question of Life: The Warnock Report on Human Fertilisation and Embryology* [*1984*], Basil Blackwell, Oxford.

Warnock, M. (1987), 'Do human cells have rights?', *Bioethics*, 1.1 [citation from Harris 1990].

Wazaki, H. (in press), 'Multiplicity of identity through urban festival'. In A. Cohen and K. Fukui (eds), *The Age of the City*, Edinburgh University Press, Edinburgh.

Weedon, C. (1987), *Feminist Practice and Poststructuralist Theory*, Basil Blackwell, Oxford.

Weiner, A. B. (1976), *Women of Value, Men of Renown: New Perspectives in Trobriand Exchange*, University of Texas Press, Austin.

Weiner, A. B. (1979), 'Trobriand kinship from another view: the reproductive power of women and men', *Man* (N.S.), 14, 328−48.

Weiner, A. B. (1983), ' "A world of made is not a world of born": doing kula in Kiriwina'. In J. W. Leach and E. R. Leach (eds), *The Kula. New Perspectives on Massim Exchange*, Cambridge University Press, Cambrige.

Weiner, J. F. (1987), 'Diseases of the soul: sickness, agency and the men's cult among the Foi of New Guinea'. In M. Strathern (ed.), *Dealing with Inequality: Analysing Gender Relations in Melanesia and Beyond*, Cambridge University Press, Cambridge.

Weiner, J. F. (1988), *The Heart of the Pearlshell: The Mythological Dimension of Foi Sociality*, University of California Press, Los Angeles & Berkeley.

Werbner, P. (1990), *The Migration Process: Capital, Gifts and Offerings among British Pakistanis*, Berg, Oxford.

Werbner, R. P. (in press), 'Trickster and the eternal return: self-reference in West Sepik world renewal'. For Symposium, B. Juillerat (ed.), *The Mother's Brother is the Breast: Ritual and Meaning in the West Sepik*, The Smithsonian Institute, Washington DC.

Williams, R. (1961) [1958], *Culture and Society, 1780−1950*, Penguin, London.

Williams, R. (1985) [1973], *The Country and the City*, The Hogarth Press, London.

Wilson, K. G. (1988), *Technologies of Control. The New Interactive Media for the Home*, University of Wisconsin Press, Madison.

Wojtas, O. (1991), 'Sir Peter exits scorning "cheap and nasty" ethos', Report, *The Times Higher Education Supplement*, 5 April 1991.

Wolfram, S. (1987), *In-laws and Outlaws. Kinship and Marriage in England*, Croom Helm, London.

Wyver, J. (1990), [Transcript] *Signs of Life*, Horizon, BBC, 11 June 1990.

Yang, M. M. (1989), 'The gift economy and state power in China', *Comparative Studies in Society and History*, 31, 25−54.

Yates, P. (1988), 'Negotiating life texts: youth, ethnicity and cultural production'. Paper delivered to Association for Social Anthropology Conference, London.

Yeatman, A. (1983), 'The procreative model: the social ontological bases of the gender-kinship system', *Social Analysis*, 14, 3−31.

Yoshimoto, M. (1989), 'The postmodern and mass images in Japan', *Public Culture*, 1, 8−25.

Yoxen, E. (1983), *The Gene Business: Who Should Control Biotechnology?*, Pan Books and Channel Four Television, London.

INDEX